Driven to be Free

Food Addictions and Unhealthy Lifestyles

By Lisa D. Piper & Amber Hackney, CSW

Driven To Be Free

From Food Addictions & Eating Disorders

Published by PraiseHim Publishing

Printed in the United States of America

First Printing, 2020

All scriptures are from NKJV unless cited otherwise. Scripture taken from the New King James Version®. Copyright © 1982 by Thomas Nelson. Used by permission. All rights reserved.

Scripture quotations marked (TLB) are taken from The Living Bible copyright © 1971. Used by permission of Tyndale House Publishers, a Division of Tyndale House Ministries, Carol Stream, Illinois 60188. All rights reserved.

ISBN: 978-0-9721453-6-7

PraiseHim Publishing
PO Box 997
Nortonville KY 42442

www.DrivenToBeFree.org

Driven to be Free

Food Addictions and Unhealthy Lifestyles

By Lisa D. Piper & Amber Hackney, CSW

Special Thanks to:

Kirstie Piper for your amazing film, photography and creative skills. We are so thankful that you are on our team!

Joanne Jones, Darlene Dakin, Mike Murrah, Sabrina Murrah, Penny Mitchel, Wendy Couch, and Paul McPeak for all of your feedback and insight during the writing and editing process.

We would also like to extend our appreciation for those who have supported us through the transformation journey of brokenness to wholeness. We love our River family and our sisters in Christ who have walked alongside of us.

Table of Contents

Every Day Matters

The photograph below is the difference that one year can make.

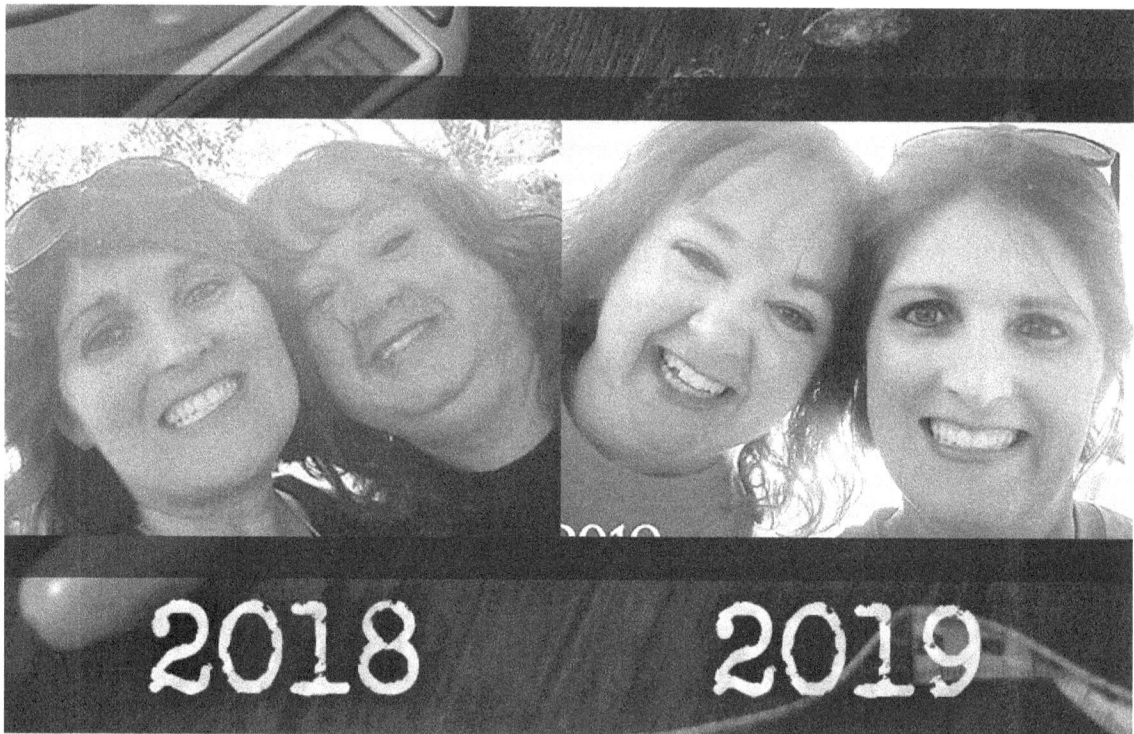

You can find more before and after photographs on the website: www.DrivenToBeFree.org

INTRODUCTION

You are reading the work of two women with very different stories who found the same answer to each of their lifelong issues with health and food.

This book is not designed to tell you what diet to follow and is no substitute for medical counsel. The worksheets and information are designed to prepare you to:

- Do what you have wanted to do, but have not been able to do (like stay on a health plan, exercising consistently, keep weight off, etc.)
- Expose any lies that keep you from success
- Arrest anything that is sabotaging your effort, and help with inner healing

Lisa and Amber have worked together on their health plan over the last two years and found success. While compiling the scriptures and keys to victory, the two decided they could not offer help to those in need of health goal support without adding information and help for those with eating disorders. If you have tendencies toward an eating disorder, please make sure to carefully read the interjections Amber gives throughout the book to give extra instruction and balancing wisdom to those with these issues.

"Eating and drinking are normal activities, but when Satan gets involved with an appetite it goes berserk: it can cause us to eat too much (gluttony) or not enough (starvation), or too much of the wrong thing (addictions, or compulsions, such as sweets, alcohol, drugs, or food fetishes and fear-motivated fixations," – Bill Banks (Deliverance from Fat & Eating Disorders/Power for Deliverance)

In this book, we will go after food addictions at the root. Are there foods you just can't say no to? Have you ever wondered why your life appears to revolve around what you are going to eat, what you just ate, or when would be the next time you get to eat? Does food appear to be a consuming thought that distracts you? Do you feel guilty after you eat or want to hide from others what you just ate? For the believer, having your life out of control when you know the life giver can be a distressing thing.

> Jesus said, "Therefore, whether you eat or drink, or whatever you do, do all to the glory of God." (1 Corinthians 10:31 NKJV)

When a person wants to obey the Word but can't seem to do it, there can be an accumulation of guilt and confusion. The focus for this work is to get rid of the guilt and clear your spiritual and emotional foundation so that you can move into consistent victory!

Lisa's Story:

I have a hereditary disposition to obesity. After miscarrying my third child in 1994, I continued to gain weight year after year and diet after diet until I reached 300 pounds. In 2009, I was able to use the Word and the fruit of the spirit to get down to 218 pounds, but before long, I once more regained the weight. After 25 years of morbid obesity, my health began to decline. I was no longer able to sit on the floor or walk any distance without having to stop and catch my breath. I wobbled as I walked. I had heart palpitations, heart arrhythmia, fatigue, and high blood pressure.

With a desperate cry to God in 2017, an answer came that removed the roadblocks of health sabotage that had marked my life.

Through the process of a group of women at our church teaming up to support each other as we tried to be healthier versions of ourselves, we realized we didn't know that food had become our idol, our comforter, our controller, our addiction! One of our friends told us that food controlled her every thought. We didn't realize sugar and carbs were pulling us by the reins and leading us into perilous territory.

Many of the men and women in this original group are involved in evangelism or freedom ministries, so it has been interesting to watch each one grab hold of the freedom we have in Jesus to be healthy!

Amber's story:

I was sick all of the time as a child and breathing problems were a scary part of every battle. I was prescribed steroids on a regular basis to help with my breathing issues. At age 11, I remember my mom taking me to the emergency room because I could not breathe. After a week in the hospital for double pneumonia in both lungs and continuous steroids and breathing treatments, the pain was compounded by the misery of my face swelling up like a painful balloon. The doctors told me my body's condition was a result of the steroids and they warned me, "You need to eat with the medications, but be careful because the steroids can cause weight gain."

The meaning of those words became twisted in my thoughts and a seed of fear was planted. My young self was terrified of being fat so I made the inner vow, "I will not gain any more weight!" Food became my enemy and the deception began to take hold. I began to tell my mom I didn't feel like eating and I avoided family meals. When I was forced to eat and given the ultimatum of at least eating toast, I would cut the bread into small pieces. If I realized I might have eaten one bite too many, I would force myself to vomit. Vomiting became easy. I rationalized that if I was forced to eat, I could just vomit the food up before it had a chance to process. Unfortunately, vomiting was not enough. An eating disorder is impossible to satisfy, no matter how hard one tries. Before long, I added taking laxatives to behaviors that were already taxing my body. I had remembered the doctors saying liquid laxatives would clean out my system, so I would take those and any other kind I could find. My perception and thought processes continued to twist without me ever realizing how much error I was embracing. Nothing I did was ever enough. I was driven to do more to become skinny because my belief was that I was unacceptable and too fat. I remember being told, "I can see your ribs and hip bones." In my head I heard, "If you were skinnier, we wouldn't be talking about your bones."

In the 7th grade, I felt like I spent most of my time in the nurse's office. I was often so dizzy when I stood up that I would get lightheaded or pass out. The nurse would just tell me my blood sugar was too low and force me to eat peanut butter crackers and drink juice. I despised the frequent trips to the nurse's station. I would argue the whole time it took to get there because I knew the nurse would make me eat and inevitably, I would have to get a plan to go to the bathroom and vomit.

In high school, I appeared confident on the outside, but I was dying on the inside. I never stepped a foot into the cafeteria and always sat in the lobby during lunch. No one questioned why I never ate, and I never offered an explanation. There were things in my life that had spiraled out of control so I was thankful that I could control one thing: my eating. I was in control of that and it gave me a sense of misplaced security.

As the eating disorder progressed, I became obsessed with eating and how not to eat. I recorded the movie *A Secret Between Friends* and watched it for content on how not to eat over and over again. I never saw the negative aspects of the movie. My mind twisted the content to see only what would end up being an influence that further plummeted me into anorexia. In a twisted way, I was on a mission to cover the shame and guilt with a skinnier version of myself; however, I was never satisfied with my goals or results.

In college, I studied hard and one of my favorite subjects was eating disorders. I lived with three other ladies and I was good at hiding the truth. I paid dearly for starving myself; I stayed tired all the time, my hair fell out, my nails were brittle, my bones ached, and I was constantly freezing. I found it hard to concentrate and felt like I had to work twice as hard as everyone else. I was miserable and hated myself. I prayed daily that I would go to sleep and not wake up. I asked God to take me out of my pain and became very upset when He did not let me die. I was mad at God because I could not fix me no matter how hard I tried and in my distorted opinion, He wasn't fixing me either.

Five years later, I experienced another trauma that left me more broken than I could ever have imagined. I had experienced abuse, shame, loneliness, and heartache, but that did not prepare me for the moment my mother passed away. I thought I was controlling food, but in truth, food had controlled me. Through her sickness, I turned to food for comfort. It became my crutch and idol. My husband is an amazing cook and I had easy access to a lot of it! To cope with my mother's sickness, I would eat before going to see her and then come home and eat my fill afterwards too. During this season, I was getting my master's degree and would eat boxes of candy while working on schoolwork. After my mom passed away, all I wanted to do was eat and sleep. I became so dependent on food that I became obese. I would tell myself that I needed to quit eating all of the junk food, but it would always be best to start on a Monday. Monday would pass and I would delay the starting date for one more week. Excuses and carbs were my friends. My husband would tell me he would exercise with me, but I didn't have the energy or drive to want to be free from my food addiction. Actually, I wanted to be free, but I didn't know how to even go about it. I wanted to be faithful to a diet, but I believed the lies in my head that it wasn't possible for me to be free or faithful. I felt stuck...like being on a sinking ship without the ability to swim.

I did not know that I was basing my out-of-control situation and hopelessness on past disappointments, traumas, and unforgiveness. But Jesus! Through Him, I found the answer and now I am passionate about sharing the truth with those who are as driven to be free like I was.

The behaviors I just described can lead men and women to becoming unhealthy and broken. Even scarier is that we can be absent mindedly led into the sin of idolatry, false comfort, addiction, false security, unhealed inner wounds, and self-hatred. Unhealthy lifestyles and twisted thinking can develop into an eating disorder.

More on Eating disorders and the Driven book: There are different types of eating disorders, but these three are the most prevalent:

1) Anorexia
2) Binge Eating
3) Bulimia

Anorexia: When a person is underweight and uses extreme strategies to lose additional weight. Some of the symptoms that are seen specifically in anorexia nervosa are hyper-focus on body shape and weight, low body mass index, and over concern about gaining weight.

Binging: When a person secretly eats unusual amounts of food in short periods of time. Even though full, the person is compelled to continue to eat. This can happen when dealing with overwhelming emotions or trauma.

Bulimia: A person with bulimia will have uncontrollable binging for a period of at least twice a week for three months or longer followed by a means of purging, fasting, or excessive exercise. Those with bulimia are focused on weight and body image.

> * Individuals experiencing bulimia nervosa also may suffer from weight control behaviors consisting of extreme dieting, the abuse of laxatives, diuretics and enemas.

Are you tired of not having control over your health? Are you addicted to any food or beverage? Are you tired of being tired? Are you weary with being out of control? Are the voices of failure louder than the sound of victory?

> The Bible tells us, " *For the weapons of our warfare* are *not carnal but mighty in God for pulling down strongholds, casting down arguments and every high thing that exalts itself against the knowledge of God, bringing every thought into captivity to the obedience of Christ,"* (2 Corinthians 10:4-5 NKJV).

God gave us power with His Word. He tells us we can allow our thoughts to take us captive or we can take our unwanted thoughts captive by leaning into His power and authority.

There's a visual that can be helpful and maybe even comical when trying to get thoughts under control. The scripture above speaks of casting down arguments and taking thoughts captive. When you get a thought in your head that will not relent, get that thing in a head lock or arm bar, wrestle it down and beat the tarnation out of it with the Word of God! Do not tolerate accusations and negative thoughts like, "I'll always be fat." Or "I am unworthy." Take hold of those thoughts and beat them to smithereens with the truth! We will show you how to do that in in the upcoming chapters!

Jesus is our Savior and He wants to help us to be healthy and He will help us to do it in the right way. This book has been designed to take you through freedom and into victory step by step. We have done our best to make it easy to understand with worksheets that will guide you through the process of being healthier, freer, and ready for sustainable victory!

> "No temptation has overtaken you except such as is common to man; but God is faithful, who will not allow you to be tempted beyond what you are able, but with the temptation will also make the way of escape, that you may be able to bear it." (1 Corinthians 10:13 NKJV)

We are overcomers with Jesus Who is faithful.

Note: See Appendix A for a note to parents and several pages of indicators of an eating disorder.

Chapter 1
Moving into Victory

Everything written in this book is going to pivot on one foundational principle and that is: Jesus is willing and able to rescue us. We are going to lean into the benefits of being a believer and follower of Jesus Christ. He has already provided everything we need for freedom and success.

The premise of what you will find in these pages is that Jesus Christ is both willing and able to rescue you. If you have any doubt, unbelief or lack of hope that He will intervene in your situation, it is best that we address that issue first. This chapter will help you look at your true beliefs concerning His willingness to do a miracle in your life.

Do not assume that you automatically believe He will come to your rescue. Sometimes we have head knowledge but not a knowing in our heart. We want to get what the Word says down into our 'believer' so that the seed of faith springs forth a good harvest. Sometimes trauma of life and repetitive problems try to ambush our faith. We can listen to the lies that God doesn't care or is passive about us, but neither accusation is remotely true. Our hope is that we can guide you into hearing what God is saying to you as you go through these worksheets.

Many confess that they want to trust in God for their health but then find themselves not trusting. Common confessions sound something like, "I do not want to overeat, but time after time, I find myself doing that very thing that I do not want to do." It is all very frustrating, but not uncommon! Take a look at Paul's lament of the battle he felt in the flesh:

> Romans 7:15, 23-24 NLT
>
> I do not understand what I do. For what I want to do I do not do, but what I hate I do. 23 but I see another law at work in the members of my body, waging war against the law of my mind and making me a prisoner of the law of sin at work within my members. 24 What a wretched man I am! Who will rescue me from this body of death? 25 Thank God! The answer is in Jesus Christ our Lord. So you see how it is: In my mind I really want to obey God's law, but because of my sinful nature I am a slave to sin.

The following worksheet will guide you through examining your heart on whether you believe the Lord will rescue you or not. Do not worry if you do have some faith issues. God wants to help you with that too! Please **DO NOT skip** this exercise.

> Go through the worksheet exercise until you have a basic belief that indeed Jesus is able and willing to help you. You may not be able to just decide that He can help. However, through your prayers, He can and will help you to believe. This work is not done in the flesh or by just conjuring up faith. What will happen as you let Him move in you is that you will supernaturally begin to know Him and know without a shadow of a doubt, He will guide you and give you what you need to succeed!

Worksheet 1: Fruit as the Remedy

Is Jesus willing or able to Rescue you?

Before we start this journey, there is one truth that must be established. Check each of the following statements that apply to you. (Pray before you answer and make sure that you're telling the truth.)

— Jesus is able to rescue me and will rescue me. He will absolutely help me.

— Jesus is able to rescue me, but I am not sure if He will rescue me.

— In my head, I know He is able to rescue me, but after praying and searching my heart, I have some doubts on whether He will do so.

— No. I do not believe He can rescue me or I believe He doesn't want to rescue me.

If after reviewing the questions above, you find that you have doubt about receiving help from Jesus Christ, the following exercise will help to get the truth into your heart. The Word is the truth and getting that truth down inside of you will help you to have the faith you need to enter into the incredible adventure of seeking and finding Him!

1. If you cannot check the first statement, then let's work on hearing the truth. Ask the Lord to make the truths in the following scriptures come alive in you: (Read each one out loud, if possible. We have an audio file of these scriptures set to music for soaking purposes on the website: www.DrivenToBeFree.org)

   ✓ 2 Corinthians 1:9-10
   ✓ Psalm 3 (whole chapter)
   ✓ Psalms 34:17-19
   ✓ Psalms 55:16
   ✓ Psalms 145:18-19

2. Ask the Lord to show you why you do not believe He will rescue you. Really listen to what He says. (If you do not hear anything right away, keep praying and seeking the Lord until you know the answer.)

3. Once He shows you what reasoning or what event has caused you to believe a lie about Him, repent for the unbelief and ask Him if there's anything you need to give to Him. Ask Him to come into every area of doubt and help you. He will!

4. He isn't disappointed in your humanity. Just be truthful to yourself and Him and let Him help you grow in your faith and trust! He is able!

THE FRUIT!

Galatians 5:16-25 NKJV

I say then: <u>Walk in the Spirit, and you shall not fulfill the lust of the flesh.</u> 17 For the flesh lusts against the Spirit, and the Spirit against the flesh; and these are contrary to one another, so that you do not do the things that you wish. 18 But if you are led by the Spirit, you are not under the law. 19 Now the works of the flesh are evident, which are: adultery, fornication, uncleanness, lewdness, 20 idolatry, sorcery, hatred, contentions, jealousies, outbursts of wrath, selfish ambitions, dissensions, heresies, 21 envy, murders, drunkenness, revelries, and the like; of which I tell you beforehand, just as I also told you in time past, that those who practice such things will not inherit the kingdom of God. 22 <u>But the fruit of the Spirit is love, joy, peace, longsuffering, kindness, goodness, faithfulness, 23 gentleness, self-control.</u> Against such there is no law. 24 And those who are Christ's have crucified the flesh with its passions and desires. 25 If we live in the Spirit, let us also walk in the Spirit.

Eating Disorder note

Believing what other people say or the perception of disapproval can lead to a personal journey of negative self-talk and a lack of self-control. Once a false belief is accepted and left unchecked, a twisting of thoughts can produce roots that aid in the development of eating disorders. Identifying the needed fruit of the spirit will help untwist lies and provide a foundation for healing and freedom.

From Condemnation to Power – Lisa's Testimony

Just looking at the fruit of the spirit in times past has brought what felt like condemnation to my life. Weighing 300 pounds certainly brought judgment from other people. I was used to strangers assuming I was lazy and stupid. When you are morbidly obese, there are a lot of assumptions people make about your character and lifestyle.

Not only did I feel condemnation from people who assumed the worst of me, I also felt extreme unwarranted condemnation from the one scripture that would prove to be a cornerstone in my future success. When I read the fruit of the spirit in the book of Galatians, the passages only added to my self-disapproval because I in no way measured up to the scripture.

I especially felt uncomfortable when I read about the fruit of self-control. I felt such shame and guilt that I professed to be a Christian yet had aspects of my life more out of control than a Mack truck headed down a mountainside with no brakes. For over 20 years I felt out of control concerning my health and diet choices. Just reading Galatians 5:23 was enough to make me feel like one big loser.

One day as I was trying to recover from a Bible class on the fruit of the spirit and self-control, I decided to pray about the situation. I prayed something like this: "God, Your Word says that the fruit of the Spirit is self-control and I don't have it. Why don't I have it? What's wrong with me?"

He began teaching me three principles about the fruit that I had totally missed. What you are about to read are principles that thoroughly changed my life.

LESSON #1:

1. The problem I thought I had was not the real problem.

I thought my main issue was that I lacked the fruit of self-control. Imagine my surprise when I asked the Lord to show me what I was really lacking in the area of fruitfulness. He took me back to all the times I quit trying to be healthy. The biggest reasons for my failure were a lack of longsuffering (patience) and of faithfulness. I was shocked to learn that self-control was only a small contributor into my epic failures.

Examples of a Lack of Patience and Faithfulness:

- When I did not lose weight fast enough, I gave up and quit altogether.
- After being faithful to eat right for a week or so, I would get frustrated that no one noticed, so I gave up.
- I got tired of all the planning and limited eating choices and opted to just give up.

While it is true that I was out of control, until I got a grip that my bigger issues were a lack of faithfulness and patience, I didn't get much headway with becoming healthy.

LESSON #2

2. As a believer, I wasn't void of all of the fruit, I was just lacking in some areas.

Once the revelation that I lacked faithfulness hit me, I instantly went into mourning. I remember wondering how I could be a Christian and not have the fruit of faithfulness in my life. It was then that He taught me a pivotal lesson! During prayer, He pointed out that I was not void of fruit of faithfulness. I was faithful to my husband, to my church, and to my children. I had a lot of faithfulness working in my favor. The problem was not that I had no faithfulness but that I needed to grow another orchard of the fruit of faithfulness in the area of my health. I learned that if I specifically targeted an area in prayer where the fruit of faithfulness was needed, the Lord would seed that area. In time, I would produce a plentiful harvest of beautiful fruit!

LESSON #3

An increase in the fruit of the spirit can help to tame the flesh and produce great benefits.

The fruit of the spirit is exactly what the flesh needs to be tamed and placed under submission. The flesh can be quite out of control. Just look at the works of the flesh listed in Galatians 5:19-21:

Adultery, fornication, uncleanness, lewdness, idolatry, sorcery, hatred, contentions, jealousies, outbursts of wrath, selfish ambitions, dissensions, heresies, envy, murders, drunkenness, revelries, and the like

Eating Disorder note

Amber's Testimony: I used food as a way to deal with unwanted emotions. My reasoning was that I could not control the turmoil and chaos in my heart and mind, but I could control what I ate. When I realized the truth of my motivation, I asked the Lord to cause me to grow in self-control, faithfulness, patience, peace, and love. He was faithful. The fruit increase produced what I needed to be released from the twisted form of control that tormented me. As I grew in the area of fruitfulness, I noticed that I no longer desired a family size bag of chips or box of sour candy when traumatic situations arose.

For every work of the flesh listed in Galatians 5, there are fruit in the spirit that if cultivated, would help resolve the flesh issue. For example, if the fruit of love, goodness, faithfulness and self-control were flourishing, would it be possible to commit adultery? If love, long suffering, gentleness and self-control were in full bloom, how could a person easily gossip?

Humans are triune beings meaning we are flesh, spirit and soul. (1 Thes. 5:23) Our soul is comprised of our mind, will, and emotions. When we become a believer and follower of Jesus, our spirit comes alive. Up until this time, the flesh is in charge and influences our soul. We are to grow and mature by listening to this new spirit man that has been connected to the life and work of Jesus Christ. As we choose to listen to the spirit of God more than listening to our flesh, we become stronger and the fruit of the spirit is produced.

The purpose of worksheet #2 is to identify where your flesh is out of control and what fruit needs to grow. Purpose in your heart to be truthful and ask the Lord to show you what area of your flesh needs to be tamed. Then, ask Him what fruit is needed, but do not assume that you know without asking Him first.

We have found this exercise of praying in the fruit of the spirit helpful in every area of life. The #1 KEY is to start praying the fruit into an area as soon as you realize there is a fruit deficit. It is our experience that prayer precedes change.

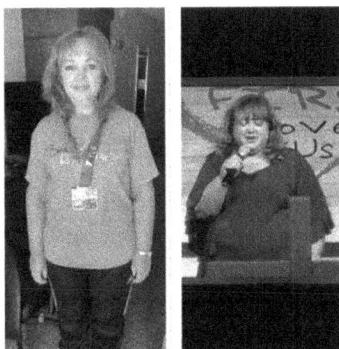

Lisa has a blog post on the website: www.DrivenToBeFree.org called, *The Fruit*. If you would like to hear more about this topic and practical uses of praying in the fruit of the spirit, *The Fruit* blog and video may be a good resource for you. In the video, Lisa talks about how she prayed in the fruit to not only lose weight but to begin exercising and prepare to run a half marathon.

For Your Consideration

In a teaching from Derek Prince called, The Fruit of the Spirit, he says the following about the fruit: *"Love—the primary form of fruit—is listed first. The others that follow may be understood as different ways in which the fruit of love manifests itself.*

- o *Joy is love rejoicing*
- o *Peace is love resting*
- o *Longsuffering is love forbearing*
- o *Kindness is love serving others*
- o *Goodness is love seeking the best for others*
- o *Faithfulness is love keeping its promises*
- o *Gentleness is love ministering to the hurts of others*
- o *Self-control is love in control*

We could also describe the fruit of the Spirit as different ways in which the character of Jesus manifests itself through those whom He indwells. When all the forms of fruit are fully developed, it is as if Jesus by the Holy Spirit is incarnated in His disciple."

You can find the entire teaching letter at:

https://www.derekprince.org/Groups/1000065927/DPM_USA/Resources/Teaching_Articles/Teaching_Articles.aspx

In the following worksheet, you will be examining your fruit and any area where you need more fruit. Just in case you aren't sure what the meaning of each fruit is, here are some definitions of the Fruit of the Spirit defined from Christianity.com

1. **Love:** Perfect love that only God can give (Jn 15:9-11)
2. **Joy:** Gladness or delight that is not dependent upon our circumstances (James 1:1-2)
3. **Peace:** life without conflict, as well as wholeness and harmony with God and others. A life of peace is safe and secures both physically and mentally. (Romans 8:6; Jn 16:33)
4. **Longsuffering:** patience, endurance, constancy, steadfastness, perseverance, and slowness in avenging wrongs. (1 Tim 1:16; Eph 4:1-2)
5. **Kindness:** moral goodness, integrity, usefulness, and benignity (Romans 2:4)
6. **Goodness:** uprightness of heart and life, goodness, and kindness (2 Thessalonians 1:11)
7. **Faithfulness:** a character trait that combines dependability and trust based on our confidence in God and His eternal faithfulness. (2 Thessalonians 1:11)
8. **Gentleness:** Meekness (Matthew 11:29)
9. **Self-Control:** ability to control one's body and its sensual appetites and desires – physically and mentally – through the power of the Holy Spirit. (Galatians 5:16)

The descriptions above were gleaned from an article from Christianity.com:
https://www.christianity.com/wiki/holy-spirit/what-are-the-fruits-of-the-spirit.html

Fruit of the Spirit Exercise   Galatians 5:22

Your second assignment is to pray and be truthful to yourself in the areas where you feel like you DO what you don't want to do and you do NOT do want you want. Ask the Lord to help you choose what to tackle first. You do not have to pick out more than one area of need, but there's room for up to three on this sheet. (Let God help you pick!)

COLUMN 1: (below) Make a list of things that you do but don't want to do or things you don't want to do but find yourself doing.   (Use a separate sheet to record multiple issues.)

COLUMN 2: Look at each of the fruit of the spirit listed. Prayerfully consider what fruit you're lacking that if you had more of it, you would be less likely to possess the problematic behavior.

Love   Gentleness   Peace

PATIENCE   Faithfulness   Self-Control

JOY   Goodness   Kindness

Your Current Behavior/Issue	Fruit Application Needed
Example: "I binge eat when I am angry."	Gentleness, self-control, faithfulness, peace, love

Now that you know the fruit that needs to be cultivated, begin praying. Even if you do not want to change right now, all you need to do is move in faith just by praying.

Sample Prayer: Lord, I have not been able to help myself and I confess that I need Your guidance and power to make changes. I desire to want to obey Your Word and be all You've designed me to be. I want to be fruitful in every area. I ask that you increase me in the fruit of (list fruits you noted.) Grow an orchard of this fruit in my life in Jesus' name. Thank you!

Begin praying in the fruit every day. As your orchard begins to grow, water it with the Word and fertilize it with action!

Notes:

Chapter 3 - Why Didn't I?

Basil yo-yo dieted his way to 325 pounds. In his library, he has dozens of books on fad diets, and nutrition and exercise videos to prove that he really has thought about his health. At 50 years old, he has repeatedly lost weight only to quickly regain again. His health is declining, and his mobility is decreasing.

Chrissy has been a diabetic for three years. She wants to eat right and knows she should, but she continually cannot refuse sugary sweets. Lately, she just doesn't even try to fend off the temptations. If offered a donut, she simply eats it knowing that she can adjust her sugar level with medication later.

Thelma has made plans to become healthy yet with each effort the stress becomes so bad that she easily slips back into comfort eating. The guilt is overwhelming...which causes her to nurse her emotions with carbs and salt.

The problem isn't really knowing how to be healthy as much as actually going about doing the things it takes to get there. We can pray in the fruit and the answer to that prayer will truly produce a miracle in our lives. However, there is a renewing of the mind, taming of the will, and a willingness to be truthful with yourself that will be necessary for consistent success.

The following worksheet is designed to help you take an inventory of what was really going on in the past so that you can make changes for the future!

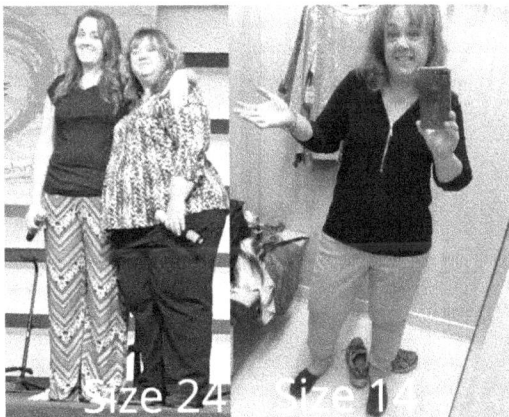

(L) Kirstie & Lisa on stage (R) Lisa trying on clothes

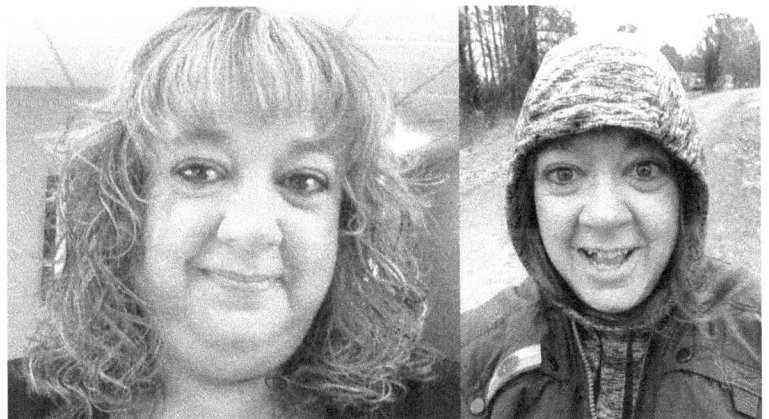

(L) Lisa at work (R) Lisa working out

Worksheet 3 - Why Did I?

Inspecting the Foundation - Psalm 139

It is important to know why you have not been able to stay on a good health plan. Be truthful with yourself and check all that apply to identify the true reason(s): (use your answers to help process lies and issues in the upcoming worksheets)

Issues with Vision

— I think it will be too difficult

— The job looks like it's too big

— It will take too long to get success

Issues with Information

— I do not know how to be healthy

— I do not know how to stay on a plan

Issues with the Will

— I don't need to change. I'm happy where I am
   o   There is still hope even if you do not want to change. If you can muster the will to just want to submit your will to God, He can intervene. I knew a man who was addicted to nicotine and liked it. He said to God, "I don't want to quit smoking, I like smoking. I'm not going to stop smoking. But, if you want me to quit, you're going to have to take it." God did. That night.
   o   Do you remember the man who had the infirmity for thirty-eight years? (John 5) Isn't it interesting that when Jesus talked to the sick man, He asked him if he wanted to be made whole. The man gave an excuse that no one was there to put him in the pool. Jesus did not ask him if he had a way to be made whole but if he wanted to be made whole. It's important to submit our wills to God!
   o   Will you be made healthy?

— I know what it takes to change, but I have not been willing to do what it takes to get there.

Issues with Hope

— It's too late to change.

— I doubt change is possible.

— I am not sure God will help me or if He cares about this.

— I want an easy way. Show me the easy way and I'm in.

— I know how to be healthy. I just do not want to do what it takes to be healthy.

— I don't care anymore. I can just stay the way I am.

— My family traits are unhealthy or obese and the hope to be any different doesn't exist.

— Change will cost too much money.

Issues with Fear

— I do not want to fail. It's better to not start than to start and fail.
— I have tried before and failed. I just do not want to try.
— Fear of being hungry
— Fear of unwanted attention

Issues with Misplaced perfection

— I'm too impatient. I want results now or I can't or won't start.
— If I can't get everything together and do it the way it needs to be done, I just won't start at all.

Issues with rebellion OR control

— No one is going to tell me what I can and cannot eat.
— I have believed that it was weight I just needed to lose and not that I needed to become healthy. At the first sign of a stall or plateau, I gave up.
— If I mess up by taking one bite of something, (sometimes no matter if it is good or not), I end up eating the whole thing.

Reasons I cheat:

A woman made a commitment to give up eating high carb foods including sugar and breads. She made it for a couple of weeks then she had a horrible argument with someone for whom she cared. She cried out, "I'm so mad, I think I'm going to get a piece of bread and eat it!"

On hindsight, what does bread or eating have to do with coping with anger or troublesome emotions? The reasons to cheat seem to be acceptable in the heat of the moment, but ridiculous later. Finding out why you cheat and addressing the issues will help you to not cheat in the future!

Check any of these that apply to you or add your own reasons for giving up and checking out on health choices:

— Self-gratification
— No Self-Control
— Physical Problems or medication issues
— Emotional Stress
— Response to rejection, hopelessness, pain, frustration, insecurity, anger, pain
— Boredom
— Failure to meal prep and end up grabbing something handy but not good for me
— "No one will see me."
— No ability to eat in moderation
— Patterns of bad eating times/patterns not broken
— Late night eating, eating too much when watching TV, binging
— When the craving comes for certain foods, I cannot resist the uncontrollable urges to indulge.
— No support

— When I fail, I just give up altogether
— I start thinking about a certain food and I eat it.
— When I see commercials or other people eating unhealthy things or portions, temptations come that I cannot resist.
— I can't say no to: _____
— I'm not patient. I want to be healthy now and if I don't get results quickly, I just quit.
— Social or peer pressure
— Birthdays
— Family culture or pressures to overindulge
— Don't want to hurt people's feelings by saying no
— Eating to please someone else or to not displease someone else
— Comfort eating. I eat when I'm sad, happy, worried or otherwise emotionally stressed.
— Addicted to sugar
— Addicted to salt or carbs
— Addicted to _____
— I get to thinking about compromise and give in to thoughts such as:
    o A little bit of what I shouldn't eat won't hurt me.
    o I did a good job this long; I deserve a treat or break.
    o If I don't eat this, someone else will get it and I won't get any.
    o If I stay fat, I will be able to hide and no one will notice me.
    o This one pound isn't a big deal. I can take it off again.

Hebrews 12:1-4 NKJV

"Therefore we also, since we are surrounded by so great a cloud of witnesses, let us lay aside every weight, and the sin which so easily ensnares us, and let us run with endurance the race that is set before us, 2 looking unto Jesus, the author and finisher of our faith, who for the joy that was set before Him endured the cross, despising the shame, and has sat down at the right hand of the throne of God. 3 For consider Him who endured such hostility from sinners against Himself, lest you become weary and discouraged in your souls. 4 You have not yet resisted to bloodshed, striving against sin."

On the webpage, www.DriventobeFree.org, you can hear Lisa's no cheat policy and how she has been able to maintain balance with not cheating. You will need to make your own plan of what you will and will not do in this journey. Examine your vision and goals, while seeking the Lord on what you need to do or let Him do to keep you from giving up in the middle of the "race."

The areas in this worksheet that you flagged need to become points of prayer. Use them in future worksheets to find out why you have had issues in each area.

Chapter 4
Twisted Thinking

Hebrews 4:11-13 NKJV

> "Let us therefore be diligent to enter that rest, lest anyone fall according to the same example of disobedience. 12 For the word of God is living and powerful, and sharper than any two-edged sword, piercing even to the division of soul and spirit, and of joints and marrow, and is a discerner of the thoughts and intents of the heart. 13 And there is no creature hidden from His sight, but all things are naked and open to the eyes of Him to whom we must give account."

Nothing will sabotage your joy or keep you from contentment like having skewed vision and dull hearing. There are women who think they're ugly or fat and they're not. There are men who think no one loves them and that they're unworthy when the Word is pretty plain about their value.

When we do not allow the Word of God to cut out every false belief, it will be difficult to walk in health, let alone have victory in other areas of our lives. We must let the truth do its work to set us free by letting it root in us.

When what we think we know is contaminated by a twisting of the truth, it produces false identity. When we believe a lie about who we are, it will affect our behaviors and our future!

Think about this! When you think you know the truth, but you only know a part of it or a twisted version of it, you will likely:

— Not receive instruction or correction
— Respond inappropriately to others
— View yourself and others incorrectly
— Not be free (it's the truth that sets a person free)
— Make poor decisions
— Make mistakes
— Hide in shame
— Be more negative
— Be judgmental

We see the effects of twisted thinking as early as Adam and Eve when the serpent used the words God had said and twisted the meaning to trick the first man and woman. If a man who walked with God and knew Him face to face could fall for a bold-faced and ridiculous lie, it is conceivable that we could too!

Nothing is as exasperating to deal with as someone whose opinions, experiences, and belief system is tainted with twisted thinking. There's a man in our county who believes he has been directed by God to do some pretty dangerous things. There's no scriptural support for what he is doing, his pastor does not support what he is doing, and no matter who tries to talk some sense into him, he gets belligerent and says, "Who am I to not do what God has told me to do!" The Word says that we will know the truth and the truth will set us free. John 8:31-32. In this man's pride, he believes he has a corner on truth and that God would make an exception and go against His Word. No, that does not happen.

Twisted thinking is often the original seed that produces a bad root. Therefore, it is imperative we deal with the twisting first before moving forward in the following chapters where we will address rotten roots.

Why is it important to know the truth about ourselves? Because how you think about yourself is typically what you will be or how you will act. (Proverbs 23:7). At times, we are our own worst critic and we sabotage our inner healing.

A woman who feels ugly and thinks she is unworthy may behave in ways to convince herself and others that what she feels is untrue. Haven't you seen a young girl who is craving attention from her father cling to any boy who will make her feel like she is wanted? Rejection can sling shot a person into grabbing onto anything that looks like acceptance.

Eating disorders stem from self-rejection and twisted thinking. A five-foot four girl who weighs 98 pounds can look in the mirror and see fat. A woman who has lost 100 pounds yet still has 40 to lose can look in the mirror and only see loose skin and fat and not all that she has accomplished. A girl with a cute nose and ears can look in the mirror and loath her features.

When we are focused on false perceptions of ourselves and not on truth, we will not give God the praise He deserves. We become consumed with our own selves which, in turn, will rob us of peace.

As stated earlier, the twisted views we have will taint everything around us including our relationships and communication. Haven't you been in a conversation with a person and they twist what you say? For example, a husband asks his wife, "Are you going to wear that outfit to dinner?" What she hears is, "I'm fat and he thinks I'm ugly. He is ashamed to be seen with me!" He did not say any of that! Maybe there's a stain on the blouse? Maybe he has no tact or likes a different shirt? We can make a habit of spinning simple sentences into twisted perceptions. Have you noticed that when we do that, we always turn what people do into something that hurts us?

If we do not reject the accusations and lies, the twisted thinking seeds can embed in us and produce an orchard of lies in our lives.

Let's talk about how this processes out through perception and health. A woman looks at a candy bar. Instead of being able to just say, "No, that's not a healthy choice," she internalizes the decision through shame and self-rejection and berates herself thinking, "I cannot eat that. Look in the mirror, I'm so fat. Pathetic!" If she eats the candy bar, shame may follow because she honestly thinks she was undeserving, and guilt of overeating may ensue.

Because we are discussing spiritual matters, you need to know there is an enemy of our soul. The devil and his fellow workers entice people to sin. That candy bar can look so delicious. As soon as you give in, that enticing turns into mocking and shame. The enemy does not play fair and he uses our flesh and mind to turn on us. We have to become smarter and wiser!

For those with eating disorders, false identities embraced because of twisted thinking will cause much trouble including, but not limited to:

— Refusal to listen to the truth from others.
— Refusal for help because the lies seem so much more real than the truth.
— A hope that what is believed is untrue, but the fear that the lie is the truth keeps them in bondage.

Pride works with the twisted thinking to produce a real stronghold. Lana, a teenager with anorexia, refused to listen to doctors, dieticians or her family. In her mind, she knew she needed to not eat to heal herself. She could not see how twisted her thinking was. Everyone else could see it. She could not and became very angry. She called the doctors quacks and berated her parents for not understanding her.

There are hurting people in hospital beds right now who refuse to or cannot eat. When they look in the mirror, they do not see what the doctor sees. They need the truth, and fortunately, we serve a God who can release a truth that can break thousands of lies!

House of Mirrors

When what you are hearing or seeing gets twisted or distorted, how will you know the truth?

Have you seen someone walking around in a house of mirrors? They think they know the way and when they navigate to what they think is an exit, they discover they were deceived. Again, they start toward what they think is "the way" only to find out that they're wrong again.

The enemy throws up mirrors in our life and the only way to make sure we are going in the right direction and seeing properly is to be harnessed to the truth. Jesus is that truth. He will reveal lies and infuse you with His goodness and saturate you with peace and truth.

Not only do our own minds allow the twisted thinking, but the enemy can stick his grubby little finger in the middle of the thought process and make the whole issue of what we believe worse. When you hear the enemy whisper, it is not the sound of a gravelly evil voice. It sounds like your voice. When you hear, "You are a failure. You are never going to be healthy. You've tried this before..." there's a good possibility this is a spiritual thing, but it sounds like your own thoughts! One way you can tell that it is the voice of the enemy is that it is very compelling. It feels real, it sounds real and can fill your senses. If what you are hearing is the opposite of what God says, it is likely a spiritual sabotage.

Colossians 3:9-10 NKJV

Do not lie to one another, since you have put off the old man with his deeds, 10 and have put on the new man who is renewed in knowledge according to the image of Him who created him,

Note: See Appendix A for a note to parents and several pages of indicators of an eating disorder.

Worksheet 4 - TWISTED THINKING

This worksheet is unlike the others in that the questions are asked to challenge you on truth and your willingness to embrace truth even if it is difficult for you to comprehend. Many of the issues uncovered in this worksheet will be addressed later. However, we want you to begin to be aware of any areas where your thinking may be influenced by error.

Heart Check:

1. When is the last time that you admitted you were wrong? (You were wrong and when challenged, you humbled yourself and dealt with this issue.)

Think about how you came to the truth and how long it took for the realization that you believed a lie. Did you have a difficult time apologizing...or maybe you refused to humble yourself and apologize. What would you do differently now, if anything?

If you have a hard time admitting you are wrong, it is wise to humble yourself because pride is the root of twisted thinking. Ask the Lord to open your eyes to pride and expose the reasons you cannot conceive that you might not be 100% right in every area.

Sample prayer: "Lord, I confess the truth that Romans 3:23 says that all have come short of the glory of God. I confess Ecclesiastes 7:20 that there is not a righteous person on earth who always does good and never sins. Proverbs 11:20 reads, "Those who are of a perverse heart are an abomination to the Lord, But the blameless in their ways are His delight." You are the truth, not me. I ask You to help me to see clearly when I try to twist the truth or when I process what is going on around me through a veil of deception. Help me to quickly repent for and confess my wrongs. I submit my opinions to you for correction. Rescue me from myself. Expose pride, expose error, and keep me in Your perfect peace in Jesus' name!"

2. Are you able to take instruction without getting angry or offended? If you cannot take instruction or be corrected, how will you ever grow? (If a person becomes offended every time they are challenged, others will stop challenging them. We can avoid a lot of problems by allowing people to speak truth into our lives. Our reaction tells others if it is safe to speak to us or if it would be best to leave us in any mess we may be in.)

3. Ask someone or a few trusted friends the following questions and give them permission to tell you the absolute truth. Write down the responses. If you need more room, use the notes in the back and reference your answers with this page number. (When they share their thoughts, do not over think their answers, get angry or entertain offense. This exercise is intended to help you. Please be in prayer over their responses. We hope you want to know the truth!) Here are some ideas of what to ask:

- **Do I believe any lies about myself?** If I do, what do you think they are?

- **When you tell me the truth, do I believe it?** __Yes __No __Sometimes __I'm not sure __I think you have a hard time believing the truth.

- **Has there been a time that I took something you said and twisted it until I believed you said something you did not actually mean?**

- **Do you have any concerns about my health?** If yes, what concerns do you have?

Prayer: "Lord, I not only want people to hear what I have to say in the way that I mean it, but I also want to understand what they are saying without what I hear being twisted. As Psalm 119:18 says, "Open my eyes, that I may see wondrous things from Your law." Also, open my ears and all my senses to take in the truth. I resist the things that keep me from thinking right thoughts. I resist offense, rejection, pride, error, perversion, doubt and fear. These things must flee from me. I embrace the truth no matter how foreign it sounds to me because the truth does set me free! Lord, if there is anything I believe that is untrue or if I don't think properly, I extend to You the invitation to come in and repair it. I submit my will to You in Jesus' wonderful name!"

Now that you are prepared to receive the truth, the following chapters are designed to discover and remove any roots that are producing bondages, strongholds, or unwanted fruit in your life.

Notes:

Chapter 5
Root 1: Lies

Have you ever been watching a television show and hear an investigator say something like, "Follow the money! If we follow the money, we will find the real criminal and not just one of his lackies!"

When dealing with behavioral and habitual issues, we do not want to tackle the "lackies." It is our goal to get to the root of the problem so that we can be free! We will take the next few chapters to deal with root issues. Not only do we have good fruit growing in our lives, but there is also rotten fruit. There are stinky behaviors, bad decisions, and all kinds of attitudes that are not Christlike, even though as believers we are called to be image bearers of Jesus Christ!

Cutting off the leaves or pruning the tree will not produce victory. Only getting down and finding out where the wild weeds are coming from and ripping out every shred of the bad root system will permanently rid us of bad fruit. Consider how a dandelion grows. A yard can be mowed on Monday, and before the grass has time to get taller, wild dandelions are blooming everywhere. The lawn owner can keep mowing over this tenacious plant, but to prevent its return, the root will have to be removed.

In this chapter, we are going to discuss ways to track down behaviors and thought patterns by getting to the lie root. We are going to follow the lie, disassemble the deception, pull out the root and ask the Lord to put in the truth.

Let's look at one root, that if left to grow, will certainly cause a horrible painful crop of rotten fruit:

> Hebrews 12:14-15 NKJV
>
> Pursue peace with all *people,* and holiness, without which no one will see the Lord: [15] looking carefully lest anyone fall short of the grace of God; lest any **root of bitterness springing up cause trouble**, and by this many become defiled;

A root of bitterness can be the cause of a bitter attitude and a mean disposition. Hebrews 12 describes how a bitter root can spring up and make many defiled. In 2 Kings 4:38-41, one of the chefs put some wild gourds into the soup pot. The prophets eating the stew tasted their supper and declared, "There is death in the pot!" When there is a bitter root, there is death in the pot! By permitting a bad root to seed and grow, there is not a part of you that will not become entrenched in the rottenness from a defiling root. Unless we treat the root, we are only dealing with the rotten fruit. Let's expose the deep root and allow Jesus to remove it once and for all. Once you remove the bad root, the areas where you really want to grow will flourish.

Many damaging roots are initially caused by the person believing and holding onto a lie. Let's look at this diagram to get a better understanding of the potential cycle of a "lie" root:

A lie is like a seed. If it falls onto concrete and doesn't take root, then the seed just dies.

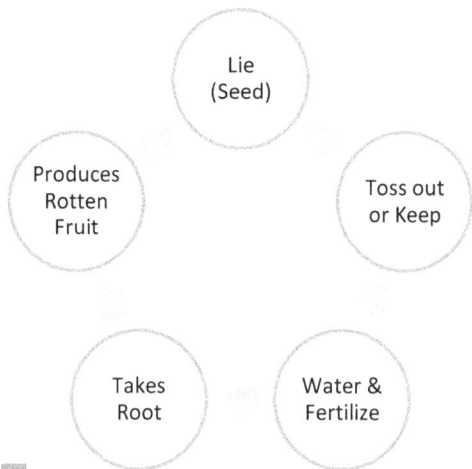

Eating Disorder note

The strength of an eating disorder is the number of lies entrenched in the thinking. If the lie roots can be exposed and the remedy of the truth applied, a healing process can begin. Consider what lies may be believed by someone with an eating disorder, such as:

I'm unloved and unworthy.

Not eating or food is the only thing I can control.

I'm unacceptable.

I'm undesirable.

However, if it gets into good soil, it will begin to sprout. The soil is your belief system. By mentally "tossing out" the lie, it will keep it from taking root, but the moment you believe the lie, that is the fertile soil it will need to begin sprouting.

Sally Mae has a father who is a bitter man and once said to his little girl, "You are ugly." If Sally Mae would have refused to believe what he had said, the seed of his words would not have been permitted to sprout and grow. However, because she was innocent and believed what her daddy said, the seed sank into her heart where it began to sprout.

When Sally Mae went to school, a little boy looked at her and said, "You are ugly." The already sprouting seed was watered with his words and the tiny little root sunk a little deeper. The rejection and lie began to get a grip on her until a bad fruit was produced. Shame and rejection bud and bloom. Sally Mae developed a hatred for her appearance and hated to look in the mirror. Because of the past root, when the lie that she is unworthy and unwanted comes, it is easy for her to believe and the stronghold in her mind imprisons her.

The process of seed planting, watering, rooting and producing continues until Sally Mae doesn't even remember what started this whole process in the first place.

In order to get to the root of a lie, we will need to do a deception inspection! Don't be fooled, if a seed is sown, there will be some kind of fruit!

Galatians 6:7 NKJV

Do not be deceived, God is not mocked; for whatever a man sows, that he will also reap.

While doing this chapter's worksheet, you will ask the Lord to reveal to you any lies that you believe. (If you knew you believed a lie, you wouldn't believe it! Because of the nature of deception, you will need the Lord to supernaturally reveal to you your core beliefs. He really does know everything about you and every thought! He knows what lies you believe and will be very involved in setting you free from them!)

Some of the lies may be as simple as, "I don't believe I deserve to be healthy," to "I am a bad person." I could list pages of lies, but there's no telling what wrong thoughts you have down in your belief system until the Lord shines His light in there and shows you what's hidden and twisted. Jesus said in Matthew 7:7-8:

"Ask and you shall receive, seek and you shall find, knock and it shall be opened." NKJV

It is as simple as asking and listening for Him. He doesn't want us to believe the lies about ourselves. He wants us to live victorious through Him! As you go through this process, you will likely become a lover of the truth because whom the Son sets free is free indeed! (John 3:36)

Before we start the worksheet, we need to discuss the issue of triggers. A trigger is a doorway to a memory. A trigger can be a smell, taste, picture, sound or even touch that takes you back to the past. When the trigger is tripped, it can bring on an avalanche of emotions or behaviors that a person does not typically express.

For example, in the example of Sally Mae, her father told her she was ugly while he was working on his car. He smelled like grease and his hands had grease on them. At the age of 25 years old, she walked into a garage happy to be able to purchase new tires. However, as soon as she smelled the grease, an overwhelming feeling of shame and an instinct to hide her face took over her senses. She did not know why and joked later that she must have a phobia of grease and grime. What she does not realize is that she has stumbled upon a trigger that links her back to that memory that needs to be healed.

When processing the lie that needs to be broken, the Lord will heal the memory and remove the trigger so that the doorway and memory are no longer attached. When Sally Mae asked the Lord to show her why she was so painfully shy and why she hated to look in the mirror, He brought up the memory of her father. She forgave her dad and renounced the lie that she believed. The Lord revealed the truth and the result was that Sally Mae no longer carried shame, the wounds, or the rotten fruit that came out of the exposed root. She chose to believe the truth and the lies shattered.

Hearing From God

When you ask God to show you something, it is possible that He will remind you of a memory. He may even show you a picture or what looks like a video in your head. He knows how to talk to you, so just ask and listen. If you ask and there is no response, then move on after a moment. It may be that He wants you to wait for an answer until you are ready to deal with an issue. Trust He knows you and knows how to communicate because He does.

A trigger can often let you know that there are some issues that you need to hand over to the Lord. Keep an eye out for things that make you act like you don't really want to act. One woman I know was terrified of cotton balls. I know it seems odd, but when the Lord showed her why, He healed her and removed the trigger. She can now touch them without freaking out. Another woman was terrified of being abandoned by her loving husband anytime she could not see him in a store. The root turned out to be that she was abandoned by her father and others as a little girl. She began to believe that everyone would leave her. Once the lie was exposed and she gave all the disappointment to the Lord, He removed that trigger and brought the couple peace!

NOTE: There will be worksheets coming that focus on forgiving those who have wronged you. Unforgiveness ties a person to the past. Just because we forgive someone, does not mean that what the person did was okay. It only means that we hand over their offense to God and cancel out the debt the person has toward us. This act then frees God up to deal with the issue on His terms. Forgiving is very freeing. As believers, we are instructed to forgive. This isn't a suggestion but a notice that we must forgive if we are to be forgiven. Please note that if you do not know how to forgive, just simply tell the Lord your heart and ask Him to help you. He will. You won't be as free as Jesus plans for you to be if you have one hand in His and one hand holding all of the offenses that have been done to you. Be healed. Be whole...let the past go.

Matthew 6:14-15 NKJV

"For if you forgive men their trespasses, your heavenly Father will also forgive you. 15 But if you do not forgive men their trespasses, neither will your Father forgive your trespasses.

As rotten fruit is a magnet for gnats, unforgiveness is like a magnet for the enemy. Unforgiveness is actually the open door for all kinds of spiritual assault against Christians. Matthew 18:21-35 is an important scripture to read and seriously consider.

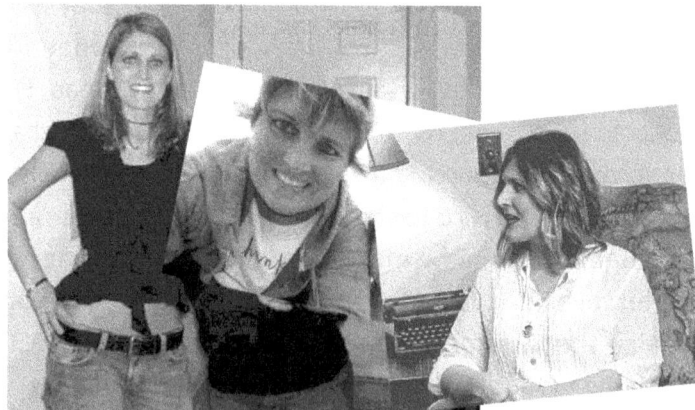

The photographs above depict Amber in three different stages.

1. Trauma had led her into a life of anorexia. (far left)
2. More trauma turned into binging and more unhealthy choices. (middle)
3. The third picture is Amber healed and whole doing an interview for DrivenToBeFree.org (Healing included forgiving herself and others while allowing Jesus to do what He said He came to do in Luke 4:18!)

Worksheet 5 - Fruit and the Root (Lies)

Locating the **ROOTS** of Unresolved Issues.

God has a way of revealing the root nature of our sins and shortcomings. For example, in 1 Timothy 6:10, we find that there are roots of all kinds of evil when a person is greedy and loves money. A harvest never comes without a seed first being planted and rooted. Our task now is to not look at the blossoms or the fruit but at the root of why we have not been able to overcome in any given area.

We are going to do some exercises in an effort to get to the root. The first focus will be exposing any lies. Please fill out the following chart: (continue praying in the fruit from the first worksheet as you work on the root section)

1: There are a couple of ways to start. You can look at worksheet #2 and grab an issue that you wrote down there in the first column and work that out. Or, you can ask the Lord what issue He would like you to work on first and write that down!   (If you cannot think of an issue, simply go to #2 and ask the Lord to show you any lie that you believe that He wants to tear down.) Here is a sample prayer: "Lord, I give you access to me right now. No matter how much it hurts, I want to be healed. Show me what you want to show me."

    Issue:

2: Ask the Lord to show any lies that you believe that keep you from getting victory from this issue. Write down what you hear or see no matter if you can believe it is a lie or not.

_____

_____

_____

3: Ask the Lord where did you get that seed (the lie?) The Father is an excellent communicator! You may hear Him speak, but more than likely, it will not be an audible voice. Listen. You may suddenly remember something someone said, you may get a picture in your head or a memory may flash back. If He does not bring anything to your mind, then you can move to the next question.

_____

_____

_____

4: Ask the Lord if there's anything you need to repent of, forgive, or release to tear down the lie. Here's how I pray, "Lord, would you shine your light in me and reveal anything I need to repent of, forgive or release to tear down this lie. I ask in Jesus' name!" Again, He will likely just bring names, incidents, or memories to your mind. When you think of it, forgive, repent or just give the matter to Jesus. It does not matter who or what you hear, write it down and give it to God.

(Sometimes people feel guilty for having to forgive people they love or who have been deceased. If this is the case, not only forgive the person but also release the guilt to the Lord.)

_____

_____

_____

5: The lies you believed may have truly wounded you. You may be wounded by your inability to overcome or by what people said or did to you. Take some time to invite the Lord into the brokenness. Ask Him to come in and heal and remove the triggers so there's no access to the scars again. Write down what you know needs to be healed, but make sure and invite Him to heal the things that you may not even know about because they're hidden or pushed down deep. If you get emotional and want to cry, let it out. If you feel like pushing the memory or any pain down, try to give that to the Lord and let Him just take it instead of stuffing it deep inside. It's time to be healed.

_____

_____

_____

6: Renounce the lie. Out of your mouth, confess that what you have believed is a lie.

7: Ask the Lord to show you the truth. He may lead you to a scripture, remind you of a scripture or tell you the truth. He may even show you a vision or picture of the truth. It is the truth that sets us free. When you hear or see the truth, then write it down and begin standing on it. This is the truth. Confess it. Refer to it. Believe it! While steps 1-6 break down the lie, step 6 will remove the root and demolish the lie.

_____

_____

_____

8: Shut the door. There may have been access allowed to the enemy because of the lie you believed. For this reason, we want to make sure the access point is destroyed and that any residue of the enemy's work is gone. We do this through prayer and the marvelous power of what Jesus provided for us. In the following sample prayer, we will address the Lord with praise, thanksgiving and petition. We will then turn and give commands of release.

Sample Prayer: Lord, I thank you for showering me with the truth. You break every lie so easily. I receive the truth you have given me today. Help me to hang on to it. I want to learn to walk in Your truth and recognize any lie before it takes root in me. I accept the authority that You have given to me in the name of Jesus. With that authority right now, I break every word curse spoken over me. And I command the enemy to let go of any foothold that was taken by the enemy because of the open door in my life. I command anything that does not glorify God in my life to loose me right now in Jesus name and to not return. And I ask you, Father, in heaven to slam the access door shut and seal it in the name of Jesus.

For every behavior or issue you find, go through this process and break down the strongholds and declare the truth!

Credit Note: Much of this exercise was taught by Katy Luse at an ISDM (International Society of Deliverance Ministers) conference. It has been so helpful in our ministry that we include the basic steps here that Katy outlined.

Notes:

Chapter 6   Root #2: Shame

Concerning our health, shame can be a trigger for some to overeat or to starve themselves. Rita was a young fit woman who was told by her father that she was fat. Ashamed of her appearance and with a desire to be acceptable, starvation became an obsession. Hatred for her appearance would flare up and trigger her into controlling her food intake when she could not control how people saw her. Shame can be a trigger for eating disorders and behavioral issues. We must get to the root of shame if we are going to get rid of the triggers that cause shame-based behaviors.

We "followed the money" in tracking down lies and now it's time to track down more of the root by "following the shame."

Let's be clear that there is shame that is healthy and when it is in proper place, it is a blessing. Shame lets us know when we have sinned or done something wrong. Shame is a signal. However, after we have repented of our sins, if shame is still present, it is no longer a signal of sin but an indicator that something has become twisted and needs to be repaired.

To illustrate how shame hides and operates, think about the hideous and yet mysterious creatures that live in the deepest darkest places in the ocean. Interestingly, the creatures of the dark depths do not survive in laboratories but die when brought up out of the deep into the light. Likewise, shame thrives in the deep hidden places where only God can see. It can be a real instinct to want to keep the unsightly shame hidden away, but when we allow God to access the darkness and clean it, healing and wholeness comes swiftly! When shame is permitted to hide in the darkness, it will continue to present problems in our lives. Shame will warp our fruitfulness and provides an environment for lies to root and grow.

Beneath the tormenting fires of shame, you will find the FUEL of lies that distort our view of God, our sin, our worth, and our redeemability.

Those floundering in the sea of shame often feel alone. The truth is that our creator God is not immune in knowing what shame feels like. The good news is that what Jesus endured when He was arrested and then crucified was a hefty ransom for Him to pay for the weight of our shame. Jesus bore enough shame for all of us.

Hebrews 12:1-3 NKJV

12 Therefore we also, since we are surrounded by so great a cloud of witnesses, let us lay aside every weight, and the sin which so easily ensnares *us,* and let us run with endurance the race that is set before us, **²** looking unto Jesus, the author and finisher of *our* faith, **who for the joy that was set before Him endured the cross,**

despising the shame, and has sat down at the right hand of the throne of God. [3] For consider Him who endured such hostility from sinners against Himself, lest you become weary and discouraged in your souls.

Shame is very heavy and can often produce feelings of heaviness in the heart, on the shoulders, or over the head. Shame can make a person feel weighed down. Tormenting feelings of shame can attach itself to our identities and insecurities.

Consider this statement that would stem from experiencing healthy shame over doing something wrong: "I stole from my sister and I am ashamed of myself. It was wrong. I am sorry and I ask forgiveness." Toxic shame becomes a fertile soil which creates an atmosphere where lies can root and grow. Consider the toxicity in this shame-based statement, "I am a thief. I am bad and I am unredeemable." Toxic shame links the person's identity with the deed. We are called to have our identity in Christ.

Those experiencing shame may want to retreat, hide, cower, or bite out at anyone who gets near the cause of their torment. The emotions around the shame can become comfortable and feel normal. We can make friends with loneliness, guilt, or feelings like low self-esteem. We need to allow God to remove the shame and cut off these friendships!

Shame related to food/health.

It is not the Lord's will that you hide in shame. (Isaiah 53:5; Romans 10:11) While you are processing shame, make sure and stop to consider some behaviors related to health and food that may be rooted in shame.

Examples of shame-based behaviors:

— Hiding food
— Hiding to eat
— Ashamed of appearance
— Ashamed of self
— Guilt after eating
— Guilt for being hungry or thinking of food
— Punishing oneself for eating or for eating certain foods
— Purging
— Lying about what was consumed or not consumed
— Choosing clothing from which to hide behind

From Lisa: Part of the worksheet exercise is to locate any secondhand shame and to give it to God. Secondhand shame can come into a person's life from a very early age. I was once speaking to a group about shame when I got a clear picture in my head of a woman in the audience. She had confessed to me earlier that she had been sexually abused as a little girl. The Lord gave me a visual of what had happened to her emotionally and spiritually during and after the abuse. I saw a picture of a male figure draping a dark cape around the woman. The cape was woven out of shame. The shame was his alone, yet he covered her with the heavy garment as if it belonged to her. Isn't that the way it is with people who do shameful things? The one who should be ashamed tosses their shame onto their victim and continues with their sin. The end result was that the victim felt the shame and the perpetrator appeared to have no shame at all. As time passed, the cape began to feel like a normal garment of her own. She learned to hide under the its heavy weight. To make matters worse, after adults began to find out about the abuse, she overheard accusations that she was lying. Instead of healing, the invisible cape was wrapped even tighter around her until she finally identified with her perpetrator's shame and claimed it as her own.

I had a time in prayer with her after the Lord gave me that insight. What He had shown me was accurate; she had been covered in her perpetrators shame. Just as He had shown me a picture of the shame cape, I watched Him remove the invisible weighty cape and cover her with a beautiful cloak of white. I heard Him say, "I will never let another person cover her with their cape of shame again. I have clothed her with my cloak. She may take someone else's garment by her own choice and put it on, but I will never let anyone cover her with their shame again." After I heard these words, the Lord gave me some instruction to give to her through a visual picture He released in me. I saw in the spirit a man holding up a gray garment. I knew this was something that would happen later to entice her to take the shame once more. He was handing it out to her as if it was her choice to grab it. I told her what I was seeing and instructed her, "Do not receive shame."

Not long after that, there was a man who said some ugly things to her. What I saw in her eyes surprised me. She had been so used to living under that shame garment that it seemed to feel natural for her to just slip on another cape of shame. I said to her, "Don't do it."

I remember that she said it was hard to refuse the garment, but instead of just taking on this identity of shame she went into prayer. There, she saw the beautiful white cloak given to her by the Lord burst into flames and burn up the dark garment that the man had tried to use to cover her. She was free. There was a change in the woman and in her ability to love in spite of being treated unfairly. Healing came quickly after shame was addressed.

The power of shame or secondhand shame to torment and cause everything from rejection to depression can be destroyed with the supernatural power of Jesus!

For every root of shame issue you find, go through worksheet 6 and break down the strongholds and declare the truth!

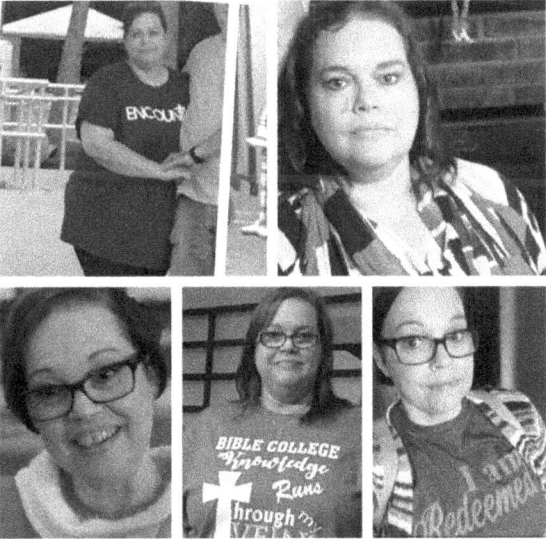

You can find the story of our friend, Tammy, on the www.DrivenToBeFree.org blog called: *Tammy's Testimony*.

Tammy experienced trauma that resulted in shame. The shame manifested in food addiction, rejection, and an undiagnosed eating disorder. After being set free and walking out freedom, she has lost 80 pounds. She is a valuable part of our freedom ministry team.

To the right is a photo comparison of the character Tammy plays each year in a children's program. What a difference a year can make!

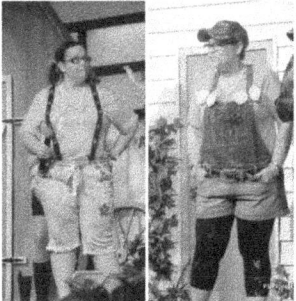

Worksheet 6 - Fruit and the Root (Shame)

Locating the **ROOTS** of Unwanted Issues.

Nothing can be as debilitating or as dysfunctional as rooted shame.

The next exercise for dealing with the root is to identify or hunt for any areas of toxic shame. The word 'hunt' is used because shame is tricky and often sinks so deep that the only one to shine the light on it and get it out is Jesus. Shame retreats, hides, camouflages itself, denies its existence and will fight to stay hidden.

This may not give you comfort right now, but there is nothing hidden from God. You can be comforted that He knows all of the shame and He is not disgusted with you. He is actually more concerned about healing you and making you whole than you are. His desire to heal you isn't because He finds you offensive and dirty. He wants to heal you because it is good for you and because He is the healer.

Once more, start out in prayer, asking the Lord the following questions and listening for His response. Again, His response may come in a picture, emotion, memory, etc.

1: (Known shame) Think about it. There may be areas where you already can identify that there is shame. You already know it is there. Use this area to write down your thoughts. I feel shame about:

_____

_____

_____

_____

2: (Hidden shame) Pray: "Lord, what shame do I have that you want to remove? I need for you to see through me to where any shame resides. Help me to release the shame to you." If He shows you anything, write it down:

_____

_____

_____

3: (Lies) Ask the Lord to show you any lies you believe that gives fuel to the shame. For every lie, process and break the lie using worksheet #5. If there are no lies, go on to the next step.

4: (Shame Processing) Out of your mouth, ask the Lord to come take the shame. Confess that you will no longer allow shame to rule or manipulate you.

Note: If you can, give all the shame over to Jesus. If there is just too much and you do not know how to relinquish the shame, ask the Lord to help.

Shame processing tool: Pray: "Lord, I do not know how to give this to you and I don't know how to process it all. I would like to ask you to translate it in a way that I can give it to you. Would you put the shame all together and show me what it looks like and then help me to lay it down at your feet in Jesus' name. I ask you to come in and clean the shame that has been hidden in me all the way back to my conception until now!"

When He shows you something, (and it will likely not be attractive), purposely choose to take that object and put it at the feet of Jesus. Literally, offer Him the shame and He will take it. The purpose is to get shame from you and transfer it to Him so you can be healed. Jesus wants to do this for you. If He shows you a picture of what the shame looks like, then make sure and ask Him what it looks like after you give it all to Him. This will leave you with a nice picture of truth and can be very healing.

4: (Secondhand Shame) There are times when people throw shame on us like we would throw a blanket over a chair. Consider praying, "Lord, am I carrying shame that belongs to someone else? Have I condemned myself when You do not condemn me? Would You show me any shame I am carrying that is not mine?"

Spend some time with the Lord forgiving those who did these things and ask Him to take the 'shame blanket' off of you. It can be healing to take your hands and remove the invisible cloak in faith. Make the motion and cast it off. Return the shame to sender!

Shame processing tool: If the shame came onto you as a child, think about how old you were when that happened. To get some healthy perspective, look around at a child the same age. What if the same cape of shame were thrown upon them? Would they deserve it? Is a child capable of carrying the weight of such a thing? No. Forgive the child you were and let the Lord heal the memories that came at such a young age.

Make sure that any time someone else's shame tries to creep up on you that you quickly refuse to allow it to root in your emotions or heart. Pray: "Lord, I ask you to release me from false responsibility and false comfort. If I am wearing a cloak You did not give to me, I ask You to remove it now and put Your cloak of holiness, purity and comfort around me in Jesus' name."

Chapter 7
Root #3: Inner Vows & Bitterroot Judgments

We will talk again later about the power we have to speak life or harm with our mouth. First, there's some work to be done to make sure we have not been the recipient of our own reckless judgments about ourselves.

Matthew 7:1-2 NKJV

> "Judge not, that you be not judged. 2 For with what judgment you judge, you will be judged; and with the measure you use, it will be measured back to you.

The words we speak have power as you can see by the scripture above. We have to be careful we don't speak words that bring judgment back upon us. As Christians, we belong to God and put our trust in Him. By pridefully making judgments out of pain or bitterness, we bind our own selves with our words. We have a free will and the Bible lets us know God will not cross our will. (John 7:17; John 1:12-13; Rev. 3:20) Through our own inner vows and judgments, we can allow the enemy into our lives to reinforce things that were never intended for us.

An example might be, "I will never be skinny again." Why even say that? Your faith came into agreement with doubt and fear which gives that statement power.

Hebrews 12:14-15 NKJV

> Pursue peace with all people, and holiness, without which no one will see the Lord: 15 looking carefully lest anyone fall short of the grace of God; lest any root of bitterness springing up cause trouble, and by this many become defiled;

Take some time to reflect on any inner vows you may have made, review the worksheet for this chapter and see what kind of difference that makes in your life!

Worksheet 7 - Inner Vows Worksheet

The purpose of this worksheet is to renounce inner vows and release past judgments that you may have made out of error, pain, or bitterness. It is important to come out of agreement with declarations that God never meant for us to make. You can set yourself free by renouncing the judgments you have placed on yourself!

Please check anything in the list below that you may have spoken or thought at time past or present. If the Lord reveals any other judgments, add those to the list as well!

— No one will love me if I'm fat
— I will never lose weight
— I will always be big
— I will not let anyone love me.
— I do not want to lose weight
— I'm destined to be overweight
— Others can lose weight, but I can't
— I will always have to take laxatives to stay slim
— If I eat _____, it goes straight to my thighs

— I cannot be consistent
— I don't care and will never care
— I love _____ too much to ever give it up
— _____ makes me big. I can't lose weight
— Because I can't _____
— I will always be big
— If I stay big, people won't be able to hurt me

Write any other vow that comes to mind:

— I will not be attractive again
— I will never exercise
— I am a loser. I'm unworthy
— I have more problems than others
— I am ugly
— I am unattractive
— I'm just big-boned
— My sister is the skinny one, I'm meant to be fat
— Being fat runs in my family. We are all just big

After you have penned your list and asked the Lord to show you any statement you have missed, spend some time in prayer. The following is an example of how you would renounce your judgment to make it null and void!

"Lord, I renounce the judgment I made that, (insert vow here). I repent for coming into agreement with that lie. I ask you to loose me from these inner vows and unrighteous judgments in the name of Jesus. I can do all things because You strengthen me. I ask you to close every door that gave the enemy a foothold because of what I believed or said outside of Your will. I submit my will to You, Jesus, and I hereby resist the enemy and command every assignment against me to release me now in Jesus' name!

Notes:

Chapter 8
Roots: Generational Issues

There are hereditary traits that cannot be changed and are passed on through the generations including eye color, nose size, leg length, etc. There are things passed down that can be remedied with prayer like obesity, tendencies for addictions, perversion, and so on.

Take a look at your family history, if possible, and you will likely see patterns of sin, sickness, and bad behaviors. Some sin becomes normalized within the family unit and can be passed on from generation to generation until someone repents and renounces the sin and its rotten fruit. It is possible for the Lord to come in and set you free from generational patterns of sin and possibly generational curses. This is important for not only you, but for your children and grandchildren!

The first step to handling the generational pattern issue is choosing whom to obey:

> Romans 6:15-17 NKJV
>
> What then? Shall we sin because we are not under law but under grace? Certainly not! 16 Do you not know that to whom you present yourselves slaves to obey, you are that one's slaves whom you obey, whether of sin leading to death, or of obedience leading to righteousness? 17 But God be thanked that though you were slaves of sin, yet you obeyed from the heart that form of doctrine to which you were delivered.

Have you noticed that in some families, it becomes acceptable to fornicate, steal, do illegal activities, gossip, or overeat? In some families, you will find repetitive patterns of hurtful things like eating disorders, early death, trauma, accidents, suicidality, perversions or even pride.

It is important that we ask the Lord to take the mask off of what we think of 'acceptable sins' and lean into the fact we are now in His family. We care what He thinks. We side with what He says is the truth. We receive His inheritance.

Rose was a woman who had suffered from the verbal abuse of a domineering and mean mother. Her mother's words of rejection led to Rose's eating disorder and severe abuse of laxatives. She was never overweight, but was consumed with the fact she might be at some point. It's plausible that Rose's mother was 'trained' on how to treat her child from one of her own caregivers.

Rose married and had her own children. Her youngest daughter was gorgeous. She was not as thin as Rose's other children but neither was she obese. While having dinner, even in front of guests, Rose would slap her youngest daughter's hand when the girl reached for a second piece of bread. Rose whispered between clenched teeth, "That bread is going to go you know where!" Rose would then glare at the girl's back side. The little girl hung her head in shame and dropped the bread. Unhealed mothers will produce unhealed daughters. The shame Rose had draped around herself was spread to cover her child and the circle of budding eating disorders continued. It did not matter how much someone told Rose's little girl that she was beautiful, the child refused comfort. She became consumed with her appearance and the unworthiness that came with all the lies she embraced.

The following worksheet is designed to cut off generational patterns and their effects on your life. It can be painful to recognize family patterns of sin or iniquity, but this step is necessary to be thorough in your healing and freedom.

There are some who do not know the identities of their parents. If this is your situation, simply look at your own life and call out issues or ask the Lord what you need to address. If you are adopted or were raised by a guardian, do not leave out any family sin by those who influenced your life.

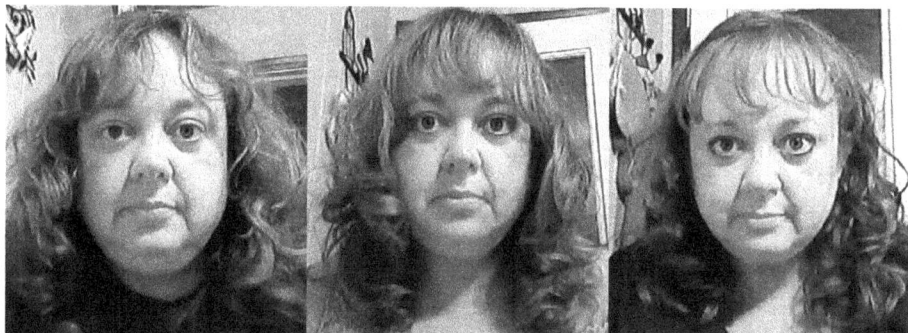

June 2   July 8   August 12

What a difference three months can make! Lisa comes from a line of women who have struggled with obesity, diabetes, and hypertension. Part of her healing has been breaking off destructive generational eating patterns. Since being set free, healed and made whole, Lisa has been able to maintain good health habits. She now has normal glucose levels and a normal blood pressure reading. Check out the story of generational patterns on Lisa's blog on www.DrivenToBeFree.org called: *Generational Surprises.*

Worksheet 8 - Weeds in the Orchard

Exposing the Weeds of Sabotage – Generational Issues

List any areas of generational sin or pattern that you see in your family. Also, ask the Lord to show you anything you have not considered. Short checklists of common generational sins or iniquities are listed below with blanks for you to write in anything the Lord reveals.

— Gluttony	— Laziness	— Suicide
— Addictions to Sugar	— Bitterness	— Perversion
— Addictions to alcohol	— Offense	— Poverty
— Addictions to drugs	— Pride	— Lust
— Food Addictions	— Premature Death	— Materialism
— Eating disorders	— Witchcraft	— Control/Manipulation
— Addictions to _____	— Lying	— Stealing
— Error	— Stirring up Strife	— Lack of Discipline
— False Religion	— Rage	— Anxiety and Fears
— Rebellion	— Abortion or	— Drama/Division
— Violence	Miscarriages	— Divorce
— Sicknesses/Infirmities	—	—
— Lawlessness		—
— Self-Hate		—

After you have asked the Lord to show you any links to your family, you will want to renounce the sin or pattern and ask the Lord to remove the damage.

Sample prayer:

"I forgive all my ancestors and those who have influenced me for all the things they have done which affect me and my life. I do not agree with my family sin and I confess the sin as wrong. I specifically request to be released from: (List all that you checked or wrote above.) I ask, Lord, for me and my seed to be released from the consequences of the iniquities in my bloodline. I ask you, Father God, to release me from any generational curse or ungodly pattern from my mother's and father's bloodlines. I ask to be released from any hereditary diseases or infirmities that have been passed down to me or through me. Please set me free from any word curses or occult activity in my bloodline. I belong to You through the provision Jesus made for me. I believe in Jesus who came in the flesh, born to a virgin, crucified and rose the third day. I proclaim the blood of Jesus as my true bloodline and receive healing through His pure bloodline. I also receive freedom from sin, sickness, disease or familiar spirits in the name of Jesus."

Notes:

Chapter 9
Roots: Word Weeds

The words you speak matter. We are created in the image of God and His words brought forth creation. In a measure, He also gave us the ability to create and that includes what we do with our voice. Some may say that we do not have the ability to bless or curse, but Romans 12:14 specifically instructs us to bless those who persecute us and not to curse them.

What is the difference in a blessing and a curse? A blessing opens a window for God to send His goodness to you. A curse opens up an avenue by which the enemy can send his messengers to afflict a person.

Proverbs 18:21 NKJV

Death and life *are* in the power of the tongue, And those who love it will eat its fruit.

If there is power in your tongue, it is important to make sure the power coming out is beneficial. Some may not believe that we can be assaulted by curses…or by the enemy. However, the whole armor of God described in Ephesians 6 is necessary so that believers can withstand the tactics of the enemy. Fiery darts are sent toward believers, it would be wise to know how to deflect them.

You may not even remember all the words spoken over you or words you have spoken that have opened the door for the enemy to come in and afflict you. The example we are going to share with you may seem extraordinary, but we know this woman and believe in the power of blessing and the ignorance of cursing.

A friend was medically documented as unable to conceive a child. After years of prayer, she and her prayer partner decided to go into overdrive with seeking the Lord on this issue. They went to a conference where there was a woman who was seasoned in prayer and familiar with spiritual warfare. As they approached the woman the prayer partner said, "This is my friend and she is unable to conceive. There are medical issues that prevent her from doing so, but I believe that God wants to give her a child."

The older woman put her hands on her and prayed. Suddenly she looked up and said, "Who told you that you would never have children?"

The Lord never forgets! The barren woman began weeping and said that from a young age, her mother had told her that she would never have children and no man would ever love her because she was fat. The grief poured out in her confession.

The older woman grabbed the weeping woman and said, "I cancel the curse spoken upon you in the name of Jesus. I renounce the curse or lie that you will not have children and I ask the Lord to cut off the fruit of this lie. Lord, I ask you to give her a child and redeem this in Jesus' name."

That was it. Tears and prayer. She went home and told her husband what had happened. After she became pregnant, they backtracked the date and discovered that she had conceived the very week the woman received prayer. Yes, our infertile friend became pregnant with not just one but conceived four children before having her tubes tied.

The power to bless is a wonderful tool. Thankfully, as easy as it may seem to speak a word curse, it is just as easy to break it. The curse began with the mouth and can be cut off with the same.

Think about the words that have been spoken either by you or others that may be contributing to health issues!

What has been spoken over you or what have you agreed with or spoken that may be affecting the healthier version of you?

The following exercise is to get rid of the unwanted roots sown into your spiritual garden that could be sabotaging your health, finances, success, relationships and life!

Worksheet 9 - Weeds in the Orchard

Exposing the Weeds of Sabotage – Word Curses (Pro 18:21)

Since we are dealing with health, we want to get healing from the words that have sabotaged our victory. Let's especially focus on names and accusations that have been spoken over us and those things we have said about ourselves.

This may be painful, but if it is, that is only because there may be a wound that needs to be healed. It is time for you to be free from the wounds of words, accusations, and bitterness.

1: Make a list of Word Curses in the chart below after reading the column instructions:

Instructions:

Column 1: Write down all the names you have been called, whether the nickname hurt you or not. If you are having trouble recalling any names you have been called, ask the Lord to especially bring the names to mind.

Column 2: Ask the Lord to bring to your memory anything said to you that is not in agreement with how He sees you. Write down what He says no matter what you personally think about what is revealed.

Column 3: Ask the Lord to remind you of everything you have said about yourself that is not true. Include in this list anything you hate about yourself or any time you have cursed yourself. I.e.: "I hate my nose," or "I can't do anything right."

Nicknames and Names	Untrue Words About You	Word curses you have said over yourself

2: As you look at the list of names, curses and accusations, ask the Lord to tell you who you need to forgive to break the power of those words. Make a list and then release them to the Lord and forgive each one. (Do not forget about forgiving yourself.)

_____

_____

_____

Prayer example: I forgive _____ for the name I was called. I release them/myself from the penalty of lying about my identity.

3: Ask the Lord to cut the tie between you and the names you've been called or word curses released. A prayer may look like this: "Lord, I no longer accept the identity I have given to myself or others have given me. I refuse to believe that I am who people say I am. I am not even who I say I am. I submit my identity to You and ask you to heal me and restore my true identity. Please cut the tie between me and every lie about my identity. Break the power these words have had over me in Jesus' name."

4: Repenting means to turn around and change your mind. Ask the Lord to reveal if you have believed any of the lies or name/identity curses. If so, repent for believing an opinion that is not the Lord's opinion. Pray: "Lord, I am made after your image. I repent for believing the names spoken over me. I turn from those names and will no longer associate myself with these word curses. I renounce the names of: _____. (say all names listed) That is not who I am. I refuse to feel shame for who I am when You love me. I renounce shame and ask You, Lord, to help me see myself only in the way You see me. "

5: If you have listed hurtful nicknames in the chart, take the time to call each one out now. Here is what to pray that will give the enemy notice to let go. (Say each name) and then pray: "I hereby command you to go in Jesus' name. Every access the enemy had to my mind, my emotions or any part of me through this word curse is to be closed right now and I command anything that came in that does not glorify God to go right now in Jesus' name. "

6: For any word curse you have spoken over yourself or if others said it, take time to pray the following:

"Lord, I renounce the curse that I'm _____. I am made in your image and you are not that! I belong to You, so I remove myself from that identity. I forgive myself or _____ for speaking that over me. I break the power this has had over my emotions, my mind, and my life. I close the door that was opened through my agreement with what was said and I command every agent of the enemy to loose its grip on me and go now in the name of Jesus. The curse assignment is broken!"

7: Ask the Lord to heal every memory of being called a name, of being mocked, or of being cursed. (Do this prayer for every curse or name the Lord brings to your mind.) **Sample prayer**: "Lord, I ask you to heal my memories and clean the wounds from names I have been called and through word curses. Remove the triggers and cleanse my thoughts in Jesus' name. I receive Your healing and Your truth! I ask that you reverse the effects of the trauma and set me free."

8: Because believing in the names and accusations takes root in our lives and produces nasty fruit, we want to make sure those seeds have a crop failure. To do that, we will ask the Lord to be released from the fruit of bad roots: **Sample prayer:** "Lord, now that I have released the words said to and over me, I ask that you redeem anything lost, broken, stolen or damaged by these curses. I bless myself! I refuse to hate myself. I receive healing in my body and command every infirmity to go in Jesus' name. I thank you Lord for restoring what was stolen from me!"

9: Ask the Lord to show you how He sees you. Just ask and write down what He shows you. If it gives you peace or joy, you will know that you are hearing properly. If what you see or hear brings shame, guilt, or condemnation, take what you heard to chapter 5 and process that out as a lie. After the blockage is removed, come back and ask the Lord again. If you don't hear or see anything, just trust that He will show you because you asked.

Chapter 10
Healing Trauma

Trauma can have lasting side effects unless dealt with properly.

Matthew 22:37 NKJV

> "Jesus said to him, 'You shall love the Lord your God with all your heart, with all your soul, and with all your mind.'"

When a person goes through a trauma like an accident, it isn't just the body that goes through the trauma, but the whole person including the heart and soul. Many times the body is treated but the rest of the person is left unhealed and broken.

It is possible for certain traumas to be the root of a low-lying issue that can sabotage your efforts for health. Psalm 107:13-16 shows that no matter what a stronghold is, we have a hope for Christ to bring us out! Jesus can set us free from every wound and every chain.

Psalm 107:13-16 NKJV

> 13 Then they cried out to the Lord in their trouble, And He saved them out of their distresses. 14 He brought them out of darkness and the shadow of death, And broke their chains in pieces. 5 Oh, that men would give thanks to the Lord for His goodness, And for His wonderful works to the children of men! 16 For He has broken the gates of bronze, And cut the bars of iron in two.

Unhealed Trauma

"So often when a person is suffering physically, people only pray for the healing of the body. But when the condition has origins which are related to traumatic events, then it is important to pray for the broken heart and not just for the broken body. The body cannot be fully healed while it is still reflecting the inner pain of unhealed trauma." – Peter Horrobin

Trauma is a side-effect of events that happen to us which are beyond our control. A traumatic event can be anything from a road accident, falling down stairs, to sexual abuse or suddenly receiving bad news. None of us can ever plan for such events and by their very nature we are always unprepared for them.

When one trauma after another occurs, a person may suffer on multiple levels. For example, consider a little girl who is abused when she is four years old and is told by her abuser she is ugly. When she is eight, a group of boys bark at her and yell that she is ugly. Two traumatic events have worked to seal a false identity in her. When she is in high school, she continues to choose abusive relationships which compound the trauma and falsely solidifies the wounds, lies and identity created out of the multiple traumas. There are eating disorders, food addictions, and unhealthy lifestyles that can stem from unhealed trauma. These problems can sometimes be a coping mechanism, or a device used to hide and cover their pain and brokenness. Most of the time, we have no control over a traumatic experience. This can leave us feeling like we need to grasp onto something we can control: Food.

From Lisa: After I was healed and set free from a sugar addiction and gluttony, I was talking with my daughter. She asked me, "Mom, how long have you been struggling with being overweight?"

To my surprise, I answered something I had overlooked previously, "It all began after I miscarried your brother, Jonah." The truth settled and I realized I had been a victim of unresolved trauma.

Unhealed trauma can not only impede our ability to have success in health goals, but the wounds can cause a blockage to our body's healing according to Peter Horrobin, the author of Healing Through Deliverance.

Worksheet 10 will take you through a process to seek healing and deliverance from trauma-based issues.

Worksheet 10 - Healing from Trauma Based Issues

Healing & Recovery

Begin this exercise by asking the Lord to show you any trauma that He wants to heal related to your health issues. It's not necessary to rehash every painful experience. You only want to listen to the Lord and follow what He says. For each trauma, you will use this worksheet to process it and give it all to Jesus. Follow the instructions after the trauma chart to pray over the issues. (The trauma can be as simple as the example listed below to a physical accident.)

Trauma Chart

TRAUMA	AGE	Anyone Involved	Any Notable Changes in behavior, life, attitude, environment, health, etc.	Memory Triggers
Twinkie smacked out of my hands and told I was a pig.	5	Father. My brother laughed.	Ashamed to eat in front of people.	Seeing a Twinkie or someone asking me if I want one.

Processing the Trauma (Worksheet 10 continued.)

Spend some time thanking the Lord for bringing you through this trauma. Trust Him to help you!

Psalm 34:4 NKJV "I sought the Lord, and He heard me, And delivered me from all my fears."

1. For each trauma listed, you will want to go through this process for healing. Start with the earliest trauma and work your way down. We are not asking you to relive every painful memory. What we want you to do is ask the Lord if there are any unresolved issues with each trauma to make sure you are completely healed.

2. Ask the Lord if there's anyone you need to forgive to make sure you are released from the effects of this trauma. Consider anyone present when the trauma occurred, or anyone perceived to be at fault. Sometimes we hold ourselves hostage by not forgiving ourselves and there are times people blame God. If you have unforgiveness towards yourself, God or people, it is time to release your hostages. Unforgiveness will tie you to the painful event.

3. If you felt like you were alone and that the Lord wasn't there, it is not inappropriate for you to ask Him to show you where He was. It can be very healing to be shown the truth about His stance during the trauma.

4. If you experienced trauma at a young age, you may need to release your 'young self' from guilt, false responsibility, and shame. Think about how you felt about yourself at the age of the traumatic event. If you are disgusted with yourself, hate yourself or feel ashamed, let the Lord come in and heal you. If you can't stand the person you were at 15, look at a 15-year-old you know now. They don't have it together…they don't know what life is. Show kindness and mercy to yourself. However old you were, let the Lord heal you and make peace with yourself at every age.

5. Repent for any bad behaviors that you blame on the trauma or that simply came out of the trauma. Own it and then hand it over to the Lord. Don't harbor shame.

6. Ask the Lord to show you any lies you believe because of this trauma. If He shows you any, go to worksheet 5 and process those out in prayer.

7. Ask the Lord to heal your memory and pull out the triggers. Let Him wash away any pain or discomfort.

8. If you need to process emotions, let Him help you do that. Don't avoid it, let yourself be healed. Some healthy ways to process or release emotions can be through crying, talking with someone, painting, drawing, writing, exercise, worshipping God, etc.

9. Finally, pray for the Lord to put any broken pieces back together and receive your healing.

Here is a sample prayer:

"Lord, I've forgiven and done all I know to do. I ask you to wash me and put any broken pieces back together. I welcome You to do this good work in me and for me. Sever any tie that I have to this incident and break off any lies I have believed. I ask You to close any doors that were opened that allowed the enemy access to me. I ask You to heal my whole self and remove any infirmity from my body. Help my body, mind and soul to heal properly. I want to let this go and I offer it to You as an offering in Jesus' name. Amen."

Chapter 11
Evicting the Weevils

Removing any seed or root that the enemy has planted is a critical part of sustained success. Jesus paid for us to be set free, the provision for victory has already been made. So far, we have covered the bad roots growing and the need for growing fruit in our lives. We also want to take a look at any aspect where a spiritual invader has come in and is sabotaging our effort. A farmer can have an orchard where the trees are healthy, the root systems are healthy, yet a weevil can come in and begin taking out the crop.

We realize that the teaching on spiritual warfare may be new to some, but this book would not be thorough without this very important topic.

From Lisa: About ten years ago, I lost around 70 pounds. I wrote a book that I thought was complete at the time. My teaching about the fruit of the spirit and growing fruit comes from that season of my life. I was praying in the fruit and seeing real breakthrough. In hindsight, the moment I stopped praying in the fruit, everything came crashing down. I not only gained back the weight but added some additional chubbiness. I was embarrassed and sad. My biggest regret was that I knew that praying in the fruit worked, yet, I could not hang onto my success.

After gaining the weight back, I just started believing the lie I would always be morbidly obese and opted to just get used to the disappointment. It wasn't until two years ago that I had a revelation when I was praying with some people who were getting set free of all sorts of bondages. Although I have seen many people set free from everything from depression, anxiety, fear, personality disorders, etc., it never occurred to me that I might have a weevil in my own orchard!

When it began to occur to me that I needed some freedom, I was so bothered by this thought that I began fervently praying and seeking the Lord. At first, I was somewhat resistant. My rebuttal to the news I had a spiritual issue was, "I don't eat all day long. I can't be a glutton. People think morbidly obese people just sit and eat and I don't. Often, I only eat two meals! You know this, Lord!"

But then He said in a still small noncritical voice, "What did you eat last night?"

I stammered, "I stopped by the store and grabbed a bag of cookies." That's what I had for supper. I had a bag of cookies. Not my finest moment. I was amazed that the creator of the universe paid enough attention to me that He knew what I ate at all times. I added to my confession to Him, "Oh. Yeah, maybe I have some issues."

I was up late that night researching the scriptures when I happened upon Proverbs 23:21:

> For the drunkard and the glutton shall come to poverty: and drowsiness shall clothe a man with rags. NKJV

I sat down on my couch and picked up the remote control and searched the following on YouTube: spirit of gluttony. I didn't really want anyone to hear me searching for this topic because it was embarrassing, but I was determined! At around 2 P.M., I found a gem.

Let me tell you, I found some whacked out videos with content I just could not digest. I was so disappointed until I found a woman talking about sugar addictions and gluttony. It was a fairly short video, but what the woman said changed my life. She said she dreamed of a beautiful white horse. It was huge. Riding on the horse was a dark, ugly, horrible looking creature. It was oozing infection and flies surrounded it. When she awoke, she said the Lord said, "The spirit of gluttony rides on a horse called sugar."

I really can't explain what happened next, but it was like a powerful truth woke me up. The visual of her dream grossed me out, but the truth of the matter made me feel like I had stumbled onto a treasure. I don't remember what I said to the Lord, but I asked Him to set me free from sugar addiction. I have not consumed sugar on purpose again. There have been some hidden sugars that I did not know were in there, but I have not craved sugar since that morning. Some people feel sorry for me that I do not eat sugar, but I tell you that I have no desire for it. I am so thankful. As of this writing, that was over two years ago. I never knew I could be free…and then I was.

About a week after I stopped eating sugar, I was driving to see my children in Lexington. I was listening to Bennie Hinn speak on spiritual warfare. He said, "The reason you may not be losing weight is because of a spirit of gluttony." You may not like Bennie Hinn, I started not to use his name because some do not, but he is the vessel the Lord used to bring my healing and I'm not ashamed of that. I turned off the teaching and began to pray. When I was set free from gluttony, I literally felt it lift off my body. Not everyone feels it, but I did. What followed later was the beginning of an incredible journey of freedom.

Later, I went grocery shopping and noticed a difference I did not even know was related to bondage. Even though I was morbidly obese, I seldom purchased chips, cookies and the like. I have always known if the junk came home with me, I would eat it. The fact I did not buy the things did not, however, stop me from being drawn to the bakery area when I went shopping. Imagine how elated I was when the 'draw' was gone. No longer did I feel compelled to go look at things that, if I consumed them, would leave me feeling guilty. I was free! I am still so excited that my cart doesn't have a mind of its own and want to veer into the deli and bakery area to take a look at the baked goods! That enticement is gone!

What a different world it was not wanting cakes and cookies. My view of consuming sugar has changed drastically. I see sugars as a doorway the enemy uses to torment me. A sane person would not offer a beer to a former alcoholic. With this in mind, I decided that I would treat sugar the way a person with a former addiction treats a drug. It helps me to say no when people pressure me to eat certain items. I do not want to be legalistic in nature, but I have a no cheat policy concerning sugar. Complete strangers have insisted I eat cookies and I try to be polite. My daughter taught me a response that is often helpful when dealing with cookie pushers. She and I were on a tour boat when the hostess insisted that I take a cookie. After hearing me say no thank you more than once, my daughter interrupted kindly and said, "Thank you but she has dietary restrictions." The woman immediately gave up and was not offended. Most of the time, sugar pushers will show understanding and back off if you just say those simple words, "Thank you, but I have dietary restrictions." It's the truth and will keep the person from feeling unnecessarily awkward.

However, if they are persistent, then I simply say gently, "I was a sugar addict and got set free. I wouldn't suggest that an alcoholic drink a glass of wine and I am not going to eat sugar either." That usually gets the point across.

I thought I was completely free and would be skinny in no time after the gluttony was gone, but I was to find that there were other areas from which I needed healing or freedom.

There are many who do not believe a Christian could have a 'spiritual weevil' but I did and I'm not ashamed of my freedom. I had a bondage and now I don't. It wasn't in my spirit but in my flesh, and I for one, am glad to be rid of it. The process was exciting. As I was being healed and transformed, I remember going up to people as I felt the changes happening in me and saying, "You don't know it now, but I have been set free. What is inside of me is going to come out and you will see change in me."

Please note that I am not implying that just because a person is overweight means they have a spirit of gluttony. However, it would do no harm to check to see if there are any pests that have invaded that would keep you from living a life of freedom and victory. Worksheet 11 is designed to help you go through the process of 'de-bugging' your orchard so that anything trespassing and sabotaging you has to vacate the premises!

Since we are considering health, it would benefit you to know the Bible's stance on gluttony. There are seemingly "acceptable" sins in the church, but really all sin is equally repulsive. Gluttony is listed with stubbornness, rebellion and drunkenness. We need to humble ourselves and rethink what we think is okay and what God says is a sin. Let's also take note that one does not have to be overweight to operate in gluttony.

Deuteronomy 21:20 NKJV

> And they shall say to the elders of his city, 'This son of ours is stubborn and rebellious; he will not obey our voice; he is a glutton and a drunkard.'

Proverbs 23:19-21 NKJV

> Hear, my son, and be wise; And guide your heart in the way. 20 Do not mix with winebibbers, Or with gluttonous eaters of meat; 21 For the drunkard and the glutton will come to poverty, And drowsiness will clothe a man with rags.

Worksheet 11 - Weevils in the Orchard – Part 1

Recognizing Weevils: This worksheet is designed to shed some light on some areas that may need to be healed or where God will set you free.

The following is a non-exhaustive list of symptoms that indicate you may have a spiritual trespasser sabotaging your victory in health. Just because you check that one thing as an issue doesn't mean there is a trespasser, but it may be something about which you want to pray. Prayerfully go through the list and check all that affect you:

I have experienced:

— Uncontrollable Craving/Drawing to food
— Fear of starvation or Fear that there is not enough
— Guilt/Shame after consuming food or not exercising enough. (like a weight/heavy blanket)
— Inability to lose weight or sustain weight loss no matter what
— Shame that won't go away even after addressing the issues in worksheet 6
— Seeking out food for comfort from:
  - Boredom
  - Anxiety or Stress
  - Depression
  - Anger
  - Emotional issues
  - Feeling out of control
  - Feelings of rejection
— Punishing myself by not eating or by exercising
— Hearing accusations in head or chatter (may sound like your voice, a voice, the memory of someone else's voice/accusation or just chaos)
— Food addiction (sugar, carb, soft drink, salt, french fry, etc.)
— Torment
— Overconsuming food/drink
— Hiding food/drink
— Buying low calorie food but then eating it in one sitting
— Needing to consume an item until it is all gone even if no longer hungry
— Trauma that results in weight gain or twisting of perception of self/food.
— Fear of being hungry
— Planning food in head when not wanting to do so
— Inability to keep eyes form looking at food, even when the desire is to not look
— Senses activated with a longing or craving from within: yearning for the food through the senses. (seeing in the mind what's in the kitchen and feeling a draw to it, etc.)
— Argumentative thoughts when trying to control eating or habits such as:
  - A little won't hurt me
  - I deserve it
  - If I don't eat it someone else will
  - I won't get any if I don't eat it now

o If I stay fat, I will be able to hide and no one will notice me
o I can start tomorrow, or Monday...or the first of the month

If you became nervous or if any pain/pressure occurred as you are reading the list above, that could be an indicator that you need to be free from a trespasser. Don't worry, Jesus paid a price to set you free and will willingly do this for you according to Luke 4:18.

Preparing for the trespasser to evacuate:

When you begin the second part of this worksheet, there is a potential of the enemy whispering a download of lies and accusations in your head. If you have a sudden overload of lies or weird excuses that tug at you and seem very real, simply speak the truth out of your mouth. John 8:36 is a good scripture to have in your toolbox for such a time as this:

"Therefore if the Son makes you free, you shall be free indeed." NKJV

Consider the following thoughts/lies that may try to take over your mind and beware of them so that you can be an overcomer when and if this tug of war in your mind happens:

— You can't be free!
— You deserve to be fat.
— You don't deserve to feel good about yourself.
— This is nonsense, fake, crazy...
— It won't happen. I won't go.
— I've been here too long, I won't leave.
— No!
— What if you want to eat _____?
— It will be back. I will be back.
— You will fail again.
— You need me.
— You are starting to look good, you can reward yourself now (and the reward will be something that will sabotage you.)

(No matter the thought, choose to believe John 8:36 and speak it out loud.)

PHYSICAL REACTION before FREEDOM

There may be no physical feelings or emotions whatsoever when you renounce the enemy. That's okay. Many times, there is no sensation. Just trust in the Lord and keep seeking Him. The proof is not in the reaction but in the walk afterwards. Sometimes people will experience sensations or what we call manifestations, but if it happens, here is a guideline for what to do.

If you experience:

Emotion/Sensation	What to do
Fear	Just ask the Lord for His peace and command fear to leave. He will give you peace.
Pain	Command whatever is causing pain to stop it and to leave immediately.
Stirring in different part of the body	Don't worry, just keep praying and command everything that does not glorify God to go until it is gone.
Lift off	You may feel something lift off. That's okay. Let it go.
Sudden lump in throat or heaviness in chest or other area:	It's leaving. Just continue to command it all to go. (If it is not moving at all, ask the Lord if there's a legal reason as to why it's not exiting. You may have someone you need to forgive pop into your head or something you need to give to God. Just listen to Him. He will guide you.)
Resistance	You may suddenly have some unsure feelings that you don't want it to go, resist that resistance and know you're almost there. Trust in the Lord.

When the weevil is leaving, you may need to just command it to go and make way for it to leave. Some people want to constantly pray. As it is leaving, just stop talking and just let it go. It isn't unusual for some to feel like something is caught in their throat or stuck in their chest. If you feel like you need to cough, then just cough. You may have an urge to release it other ways like burping, coughing, crying, etc. Don't hold it in, just let it out.

Understanding this process can be a little confusing, so we wanted to give an example as to how something could be "lodged" inside of your flesh or soul realm. Mary Jo was ten years old when a bully called her fat and said that he hated her. Embarrassed and angry, she could feel sadness and hatred in the pit of her stomach. She was so mortified that she felt nauseated. She was in front of about ten classmates. She did not want the others to see her cry, so she pushed away the tears and yelled out, "I hate you. And it's you who is ugly!" She walked away and in a private bathroom stall, she wept silently while she made the inner vow, "I won't let them see me cry and I will make him pay. I will never eat again." She shoved the unresolved hurt down and there it lodged and began to work its bitterness in her life. Unhealed effects of trauma do not just go away. A doorway was opened, and the enemy used the wound to plant rejection, fear, anger, and self-hatred. When we are getting rid of these wounds and "weevils", it can feel like the brokenness just comes out of the same place where the hurt landed.

Please make sure you have reviewed and prayed through the previous worksheets 1-11 before you proceed to this section. The other exercises serve to remove any legal ground by which the enemy had rights to trespass. Once the legal rights have been severed, then you can evict trespassers with authority.

To prepare for the 'eviction' process, we recommend choosing a time when you can pray and rest. Some people feel like a million bucks after going through this process while some people feel like they have run a marathon. So just in case, have some time carved out to rest and reflect on the goodness of the Lord.

Worksheet 12 - Weevils in the Orchard – Part 2

Evicting Trespassers: Removing the Trespassing Weevils that work to destroy.

Spend some time in worship and perhaps read Isaiah 53. When you feel at peace about evicting the trespassers, prepare yourself to just let it go and put your trust God.

The following are some names of certain enemies that may be sabotaging you. It would not hurt to just renounce them all and then pray the prayer at the end.

After you go through the list, ask the Lord if there's anything else you need to renounce and command to go. If He tells you something, write it down and renounce that as well.

Note: As you are going through the list, you may feel a "witness" or a "confirmation" inside that there is a real issue with one of the names listed. For example, when you renounce False Comfort, you might suddenly feel sad or you might feel an odd knowing that false comfort has especially been a problem. Put a dot beside of false comfort. As you read, if more items stick out to you, make more dots on each item. After you are finished with the list and have prayed, go back to the ones you marked with a dot and pray until you no longer have an uneasiness. Renounce each one and command it to go until the peace of Jesus comes.

Begin by saying, "I renounce the following lifestyles and sins. If there is anything in me, on me or around me that does not glorify God named or unnamed I command it to leave now in the name of Jesus: (begin reading list below)

— Gluttony	— Anything Seducing	— Self-Gratification
— Food Addiction	— Bondage of Food	— Ungodly Appetite
— Sugar Addiction	— Overeating	— Chocolate Addiction
— Disobedience	— Self-Indulgence	— Carb Addiction
— Lust	— Pride	— Salt Addiction
— Lust of the Eyes	— False Comfort	— Caffeine Addiction
— Lust of the Flesh	— False Responsibility	— Purging
— Seduction	— Passivity	— Heaviness
— Laziness	— Anorexia	— Depression
— Complacency	— Bulimia	— Anxiety
— Poverty	— Binging	— Fear of Starvation
— Lying	— Shame	— Starvation
— Self-Hate	— Infirmity	— Fear of Abandonment
— Hatred for Others	— Idolatry	— Accusations and Blaming
— Unforgiveness	— Unhealthy Control	— Excuses
— Root of Bitterness	— Rejection	— Infirmity
— Guilt & Shame	— Self-Rejection	—
— Hopelessness & Negativity	— Fear of Rejection	—
	— Bad Attitudes	

Pray: "Lord, I have renounced these works of the flesh and every foothold of the enemy. I ask you to cut off their power and release me into freedom. Set up your seal and do not allow these weevils or any other spiritual pests to harass, torment or try to come back, right now in Jesus' name."

(If you read the instructions, just keep praying until the release of peace comes. The process of the healing and freedom can take just a moment or it may take a little while. Just trust in the Lord and He will guide you. If you need help praying, find a believer who can agree with you to be with you. Choose someone who is balanced and peaceful.)

Now, once this is finished, thank the Lord for His good work. It is important to trust Him and write down what He has done. The enemy can come pretty quickly to lie to you that God didn't do anything or that the enemy's plans aren't demolished, but that's a trick to cause you to fear or to get you to believe his lies over the truth. It is important to believe God and not come into agreement with any lie or accusation that is presented by the enemy.

Important wisdom:

- If those lies and accusations come back afterwards, just quote the Word again and choose to believe what the Word says. Out of your mouth, say the truth. For example, if a thought comes, "You are going to fail. You won't last a week." Respond with your mouth, "Whom the Lord sets free is free indeed and I will not fail!"
- After you're finished with the prayer, just trust in the Lord. There is a course called Post Deliverance on the www.DrivenToBeFree.org website. You will want to hold your position and not give the enemy a place to try to camp out again and this course can help you! The enemy will likely not delay to sow lies, so this course will aid you in recognizing a lie when you hear it. We are very excited to know that God is healing you, making you whole, and setting you free!
- Some of the things you need to do to maintain an atmosphere of healing is stay in the Word, spend time with God, and fellowship with other believers!
- You may have experienced healing in your body or mind as you are going through this book. It is very important to not give your healing away. If a 'familiar' pain comes back tomorrow, just simply command it to go and proclaim your healing. Note that sometimes healing takes place immediately and sometimes the Lord just clears out the things that have hindered your body from healing naturally. Just trust in Him and walk it out. Grab your healing and hang on!

Chapter 12
Choosing structure/Submitting to God

So far, what we have done is clean out the foundation and anything that would make you stumble in your quest for good health! Now, it is time to do some research and make whatever changes are needed for optimum health!

We realize that there are some who will read this book and think, "C'mon, just tell me what diet to choose!" This book is about how to be consistent, live free, and remove any roadblocks to making healthy decisions through Biblical truths.m

Our counsel is that you have come this far to prepare the way through prayer, why not seek the Lord for your own health? Who knows your body better than He? We've been working on fine tuning your abilities to hear from Him and remove the barriers to communicating with Him through the worksheets.

To help you see how getting free from lies, shame, strongholds and bondages helped us, we are going to leave more of our personal testimonies below. When you mix freedom in with a good health plan, it really will help you to be successful!

> **THE GOAL**
>
> The goal is to be healthy spiritually, emotionally, and physically. If health is not the goal, when you plateau, you might be tempted to throw your hands up and quit. The goal is less bloating, better range of motion, more energy, less fatigue, etc.

Lisa's Story:

I was set free from sugar addiction and the spirit of gluttony in August of 2017. I no longer craved carbs and sugars at all. I ate until I was full and stopped. No longer did my husband and I go to a buffet where I filled two plates to overflowing. I easily just ate what I wanted and stopped. I stopped going to the dessert bar period. I initially lost a few pounds but did not keep that off. I was set free and still heavy.

It so happened that we had a winter storm early in 2018. My husband and I were in the house hibernating for a week. At the end of the week, I discovered something I just didn't think to recognize. Although I had not overeaten…nor had I eaten sugar, I had not consumed one vegetable the whole week! I probably had mashed potatoes, but no greens.

I only knew to go back through my process again as outlined in this book and ask the Lord what else needed to be done. I began looking at where I was failing and lined up all the fruit of the spirit I would need to overcome. I simply began to pray, "God, I don't know anything about nutrition. I don't know what is right and I do not want to go on a yo-yo diet. I'm willing to eat whatever even if I don't like it, I just need help."

I did not want to do just low carb because my past experience was kidney pain when I tried to increase protein. I did not want to count calories because I just didn't think I would do that forever, but I was willing! What I have found to be the best is to seek the Lord and ask Him what is best. Some people just choose healthy foods, eat when they're hungry and stop when they're full. They ask the Lord to guide them in food choices. For me, well, I needed something a little more radical. I had more than 150 pounds to lose and although the task was daunting, I prayed fervently for the solution.

I realize that my way of eating can be controversial, but it is perfect for me. A friend of mine who had been set free called me and asked me to go on the ketogenic diet with her. I told her I didn't even know what it was, but I'd think about it. I thought and prayed because I had been seeking for an answer.

Within a day, I agreed to start the plan. I didn't know what I was doing until I found Dr. Eric Berg's videos. He teaches a healthy clean version of keto. Yes, the diet requires giving up sugar, grains, pastas, cereals, root vegetables, bread, and snacks. But, without the craving and just a desire for health, I followed the plan. I've eaten more greens and veggies since I started than I probably had my entire life! Finally, I not only started getting healthy, but I lost weight.

Just because a person gets spiritually and emotionally healed and set free does not mean that total health is automatic. We need to renew our minds in the Word, fill it with truth and change habits. The change is just easier to do without the bondages and with spiritual fruit growing everywhere possible!

For me, the difference is amazing. I don't cheat because this is my life and I don't want to sabotage my body. If I were to fail, I'd cling to the Word and get back up and not give the enemy a place to shame me or trap me.

Prior to changing how I ate, here are some personal issues that I journaled:

(You will find lots of before and after photos in my blogs on the www.DrivenToBeFree.org website.)

- ✓ loud snoring
- ✓ chest pain
- ✓ heart out of rhythm
- ✓ could not get down in the floor and back up without pain and it took me a long time to do this
- ✓ muscle spasms
- ✓ itching and burning feet
- ✓ eye twitching
- ✓ right side pain
- ✓ double/triple chin

Within a few weeks, the loud snoring, chest pain, feet issues and side pain were gone. As I have lost weight, mobility has returned, and my chin is less chubby every month. The muscle spasms continued until I went through another round of freedom and the Lord did heal that issue. I am very thankful.

I surrounded myself with others who were on the freedom and health journey with me. I subscribed to some FB pages of others doing keto and I listen to videos and podcasts regularly.

I have experienced months when there is no change in my weight. However, this isn't about weight, it is about health and me being steady and doing the right things. Every time I stall, I come out of it.

Amber's Story: My victory from an eating disorder that haunted me for over 22 years came in June of 2018. I had lost complete control. Food had been my way of dealing with emotions since I was a young child. The torment started with not allowing myself to eat food and it ended with over consumption. I would eat fast food on the way to the hospital to visit my mother, eat snacks while there, and eat again on the way home. The only vegetable I consumed was the piece of lettuce on my double cheeseburger. I would wake up in the middle of the night just to eat a bowl of cereal. My thinking was filled with obsessing over food and what I would eat. I thought about my next fix and the time in between eating came closer together. I had an addiction that was affecting every area of my life. Just like no one ever guessed that I had been starving myself, no one knew what was happening with my life controlling issues.

The Focus!

Weight loss is an amazing reward, but not the focus. If the focus is only on weight loss, then when the scales show no movement, we will want to quit. If we know the roots of why we couldn't lose and the fruit of what caused us to become healthy and obtain a healthy weight, then we can just keep going and maintain our success!

One day I remember looking in the mirror and did not recognize the person I had become. I was broken, lost, and overweight. My mother had died from a rare disease at the age of 49 and I was already seeing the same symptoms from which she suffered in my own body including a fatty liver, overweight, no energy, difficulty breathing, and elevated liver enzymes. Even though I knew the probable outcome to my behaviors, I did not have the willpower to quit eating; so, I did what most of us do, I went to the weight doctor. I had family and friends tell me this was the answer. The weight doctor had this magic pill that was going to increase my energy and help the pounds melt away. Man, I was so disappointed when that did not happen. Not only did I not lose ANY weight, but I GAINED. Here I was putting all my eggs in this basket and they just broke. I remember thinking, "Well, I might as well eat all I want since I am never going to be able to do this." I went home and ate pizza, cheese bread, hot wings, a bag of Cheetos, a box of sour candy, and a snack cake. It felt so right in the moment, and then I was miserable.

The next day, I made an appointment with my family doctor and he prescribed me sleep, depression, and ADHD medication. He was really trying to help me, but medications were not what I needed. I took the medication and joined a gym just to learn, again, the scales did not move. When that plan failed, I revisited the weight doctor. I thought I must have missed something that was important for this miracle medication to work. I shared my experience and they told me I was missing B12, so they sold me a package of B12 shots. My husband gave me a shot for the next four weeks. I was working out, I started eating better, and taking all this medication, but nothing was working.

Finally, I gave it all to Jesus. In my brokenness, I boldly and unashamedly told him I was miserable, unhappy, overwhelmed, disgusted, unhealthy, and scared. I found the right answer, and just like that, He started to heal my broken heart. It was not an easy process and it was lots of work, but it was so worth it. If you have been digesting and progressing through the worksheets in this book, then you are going through the same steps that I went through to get healed, whole, and set free. I linked up with Lisa and a few other ladies from church and my life was transformed because of freedom. Lisa had decided to start a healthy lifestyle at about the same time as I did. She started a helpful Facebook page that provided some accountability too. I thought about everything I had tried and knew Keto was what I needed to do. I am not telling you that this is the health plan answer for you. The answer is

Jesus and the freedom He provides. Keto was a health choice and I was thankful to have a friend with whom I could go through the process. We started walking after church with a group of individuals and I researched different meals that I could eat. I think I should mention I did not have a lot of money and I do not cook and I do not meal prep. I worked with what I could afford and leaned into Jesus. The first week, I lost 3 pounds. This was the first time the scales showed a decrease in as long as I could remember.

I finally felt that I was getting somewhere. My strength came from Jesus, my encouraging friends, and my husband. I remember my husband looking at me and saying, "I never realized how big you had gotten until I look at you now and how much you have lost." When the thought came, "One little bite won't hurt," I knew I needed to pray because something was going wacky. The whole process of getting healthy and maintaining what you achieve requires keeping your flesh in check, growing in the fruit, and not allowing any compromise when it comes to the truth or health. Our body is the temple of the Holy Spirit and we must keep that in mind...not in a way that produces guilt and shame but to spur us on to victory!

1 Corinthians 6:19-20 NKJV

> Or do you not know that your body is the temple of the Holy Spirit who is in you, whom you have from God, and you are not your own? For you were bought at a price; therefore glorify God in your body and in your spirit, which are God's.

My faithfulness, patience, and self-control were tested when the next trauma came into my life. My grandmother passed away and I found myself turning to food for comfort. I did not realize I was self-sabotaging until Jesus had a little talk with me. He said, "You lost your faith in me because I didn't do what you thought I would do." I cried because he was right. The bitterness of my loss had transformed into weevils that were eating up my spiritual fruit. I went through the prayers in this book again and jumped back on the horse. I had no shame of failure. No guilt. No condemnation. I had let my spiritual fruit be devoured, but I was able to recognize that there was a thief trying to steal my health and I was not going to allow that to happen. Spiritual and physical health are the keys here. Not weight loss! Weight loss is an amazing reward, but not the focus.

Although it has not been easy, the Word of God has been a constant strength. Psalm 91 is a tremendous passage for remembering that we are not alone and that He really will rescue us and deliver us!

> Psalm 91:1-4 NKJV
>
> He who dwells in the secret place of the Most High
> Shall abide under the shadow of the Almighty.
> 2 I will say of the Lord, "He is my refuge and my fortress;
> My God, in Him I will trust."
>
> 3 Surely He shall deliver you from the snare of the fowler
> And from the perilous pestilence.
> 4 He shall cover you with His feathers,
> And under His wings you shall take refuge;
> His truth shall be your shield and [b]buckler.

Worksheet 13 - Structure and The Plan – Part 1

Changing habits and renewing your mind!

The first order of business is to pray. Ask the Lord to help you see areas where you could improve in your health. Ask Him to help you enjoy this process so that you aren't tempted to make it a legalistic bondage.

Simply pray about and ask yourself the following questions:

1. Is my eating and drinking bringing glory to God? (1 Corinthians 10:31)
   — When you are about to eat, think about it. Is what you are eating good for you? Is your choice a response of thankfulness for the body He has given to you? If what you are about to do is not, then why do it? (There should be no shame in your answers. If you feel shame or guilt, then go into prayer and perhaps seek the Lord about why there's still shame and perhaps do the shame worksheet again.)
2. Is what you are eating nutritional? Is it something you are supposed to be consuming?
   — 1 Timothy 4:4-5 says that what God has made is good and not to be refused when received with thanksgiving. You may want to check what you are consuming and make sure it is something that was designed to be consumed. (Genesis 1:29; Genesis 9:3)
3. What adjustments could you make that would be healthier for you?
   — Research some nutrition information and get a plan. The plan needs to be doable and long term for you. For example, eating all meat isn't likely something you'll do forever. Eating only sub sandwiches isn't really a good plan. Eating only popcorn or only apples just is not a good health plan. If you have had an eating disorder, you will want wise counsel for what you choose. We happen to like Dr. Eric Berg, Dr. Jason Fung, Dr. Boz, and Dr. Ken Berry.

As you consider and pray about the questions above, be driven to do any research needed to make a good plan for success. Be willing to study the Word, pray, and study about issues that you have identified in yourself. If you do not have the desire yet to be driven, simply start praying in the fruit in this area. God will be faithful and will help you get driven! We have friends who have gotten healthier with various eating and exercise plans. God really will help you pick a plan that is right for you!

Scale Bondage: It is exhilarating when the pounds come off, but emotions can spiral out of control when either the scale doesn't move or if reports an increase. The fruit of the spirit may need to be grown in this area of peace on the scales. It is entirely possible to get on the scale and not be moved by what you see. It is also possible to control yourself from getting on the scale frequently. It takes as much self-control to not weigh as it does to eat healthily.

The recommended goal is to:

1. Weigh without feeling "compelled" to do so. You should be able to say no, I won't weigh.

2. Have no emotional meltdowns, depression, or self-hate when the scale reports the results.

Check for behaviors during this process that can rob you of peace like your attitude after getting on the scale.

- Does the weight on the scale affect the way you view yourself?
- Do you control the scale, or does it control you? If it controls you, go back through the worksheets and try to pinpoint the root issues.
- When you step on the scale and there is no movement or you gain weight, what is your response?
  - Desire to give up or quit
  - Sling the scales through the nearest window
  - Depression
  - Melt down of emotions
  - Go eat your favorite food
  - Anger
  - No emotion
  - Invigorates you to want to try harder
  - Self-hatred
  - Self-harm (which includes but not limited to physically punishing yourself through physical pain, refusing food, exercise, etc.)
  - Other: _____
- What response would you like to have when you get on the scale?
  - Make a plan and begin doing that thing. Your emotions will catch up as you discipline your mind, pray in the fruit, and get control of your life!

Pray: Father, You are in charge of my life. I do not like it when the scales take control of me. I ask that You give me the right mindset when weighing. I give the scales to You and ask You to show me what I need to change. I ask for You to increase me in the fruit of self-control, patience, love, gentleness, and faithfulness when it comes to an eating plan, exercise plan, and when I weigh. I want my motives to be pure. Release me from all bondage to yo-yo dieting, fad diets, unhealthy life choices, and from any addiction to the scales, pills, foods, habits, or wrong ideas that I have, in Jesus' mighty name.

Take some time to think about His response. You can do it! You can be healthy. When you do the right things, it is easier to be more confident when you get on the scales. If the numbers go up, you can confidently say, "I haven't done anything wrong. I am not going to beat myself up." And if you have fallen, you can say, "This is an unfortunate number, but it does not control me. I have risen from where I fell and am a victor in Christ Jesus!"

Chapter 13 - Choosing structure/Submitting to God
(Eating Disorder Focus with Amber)

Note: See Appendix A for a note to parents and indicators of an eating disorder.

Eating disorders are dangerous and we must be careful how we handle the things that trigger us back into a place we do not want to be! Recently, while I was on a strict version of keto, I came down with a nasty cold virus. The doctor prescribed steroids. Remember what I said happened to me as a child which jump started the eating disorder? I have been living free, but when my physician prescribed steroids, I was not prepared for what my mind would do. I had to take food with the medicine, but the medicine would make me gain weight. The overwhelming decision of what to do was heavy on me. My mind went immediately to that sickly little girl sitting in my room fearful to eat because I might gain weight.

THE GOAL

The goal is to be healthy spiritually, emotionally, and physically without triggering and going back into behaviors and bondage of the past. The goal is to have our identity in Christ and not in our own image!

If you understand the fierce and speedy downward spiral an eating disorder can take, then you will know I had to immediately enforce 2 Corinthians 10:5. I forcibly had to take captive thoughts that if I ate I would become fat or I would fail on the diet because the medicine would make me gain weight.

2 Corinthians 10:4-5 NKJV

> For the weapons of our warfare are not carnal but mighty in God for pulling down strongholds, 5 casting down arguments and every high thing that exalts itself against the knowledge of God, bringing every thought into captivity to the obedience of Christ,

I began to line up my thinking with the Word and speak the truth. I was feeling shame because everyone else on my health team was on this diet plan and I was sick. I know that shame always needs to come into the light because it will grow and reproduce in the darkness. I called a friend and told her what I was experiencing and what the doctor had prescribed. In wisdom, she said that I should get well, do as the doctor said, and not feel ashamed because it was not my fault. She added to her counsel, "And above all, do not fall for the triggers that might try to rekindle the past eating disorder." I stopped the fasting I was doing and started eating healthy foods. It was plain that the enemy was trying to throw me off my game and I was already waiting for him to move so I could take it to Jesus. My point here is that the enemy doesn't play fair and we have to be ready when he tries to hinder our overall wellness. If my mind had not already been in the process of renewal, this situation may have had a different outcome.

Romans 12:2 NKJV

> And do not be conformed to this world, but be transformed by the renewing of your mind, that you may prove what is that good and acceptable and perfect will of God.

Worksheet 14 - Structure and The Plan – Part 2

This worksheet is specifically designed to process triggers until they are healed and gone. During your health plan, if any triggers hit, come to this worksheet! This is a tool for you so you will be successful. The enemy has a plan and you certainly need a success plan of your own. A trigger is just a reminder of the destructive pattern and we need to allow God to deal with that immediately.

Recognize the Trigger(s):

1. Write down anything you know that is a trigger that takes you to a place where you might fail.
2. If you are experiencing a backset and you aren't sure what caused it, simply pray and ask the Lord to show you any triggers that you need to address. Ask the Lord to show you what you need to know.
   — This can sometimes be emotionally charged. If you are feeling overwhelmed in this process, close your eyes and call upon Holy Spirit to help you. Once you are able to recall the trigger, write it down below. Note: There are some who need help processing triggers. Never be ashamed to call in a good health professional or even a prayer partner to assist.

Trigger(s):

_____

_____

_____

Memory Recall

Ask the Lord to show you any memories that are not healed that are keeping you from getting victory from this issue. Write down what you hear or see. You may suddenly remember something someone said, you may get a picture in your head, or a memory may flash back. As He shows you, make sure and ask Him if there are any lies you believe and allow Him to reveal the truth so that your identity is renewed and aligned in the truth!

_____

_____

_____

Healing

Ask the Lord to heal the memory and pull out or remove the triggers. Let Him wash any pain or discomfort away. Let Him get rid of the unwanted seeds sown into your spiritual garden that could be sabotaging your health. Do not hold back. Let his love and peace comfort you in this step. Trust Him to do the work in you.

Sample prayer: Jesus, I welcome you to come and heal the memory of _____. I submit this memory, the pain, and the trauma to You. I ask You to come in and heal anything in me that shattered in this memory. Please remove the trigger that accesses this memory in Jesus' name.

Let the Light Chase out any Darkness

Ask the Lord if there's anything you need to repent of, forgive yourself or others for that has caused the trigger(s) to surface. Here's how I pray, "Lord, would you shine your light in me and reveal anything hiding in the darkness that I need to let go of, repent of, or forgive. I choose to forgive myself and _____ . By my own free will, I release those who caused me pain."

Again, He will likely just bring names, incidents, or memories to your mind. When you think of it, forgive, repent or just give the matter to Jesus. It does not matter who or what you hear, write it down and give it to God.

_____

_____

_____

Sever Ties & Loose Strongholds

Sample Prayer: "Lord, I am thankful for the work you are doing in me. I ask you to wash me and sever any ties to triggers from my past food addiction or eating disorder(s). I welcome you to do this good work in me and for me. I ask you to close any doors that were opened that allowed the enemy access to me. Lord, you are my help and my deliverer. I ask you to heal my whole self and remove the memory triggers from my mind and thoughts. Help my body, mind and soul to heal properly. Help me remain healthy and not return to past behaviors. I want to let this go, never to return, so that I can be free in you. I offer it to you as an offering in Jesus' name. Amen."

If you were involved in laxative or medication abuse, it might be helpful to renounce the tie to those items. A sample prayer for someone who has misused laxatives might be: "I renounce the unhealthy use of laxatives. *(If you have a favorite brand, call out the name.)* I ask You, Lord, to sever my tie and desire or compulsion to use them. I renounce the lie that laxatives are my friend and helpful to me. I renounce the shame of misusing laxatives and I command any foothold the enemy had over me through this open door to go in Jesus' name. Lord, close this door and set me free from this misuse or addiction. I also ask that you restore my body so that it functions without laxatives. I ask you to heal me and make my body whole through the love and provision of Jesus Christ."

Staying Trigger Free

You will want to be prepared if something happens and a trigger tries to return. It is not unlike the enemy to be sneaky and try to make you think that you're going backwards instead of forward. It is important to replace your triggering thoughts with good thoughts that honor God. Write some scriptures or thoughts below so that you can recall them and recite them in a time of crisis: (Example: When I feel out of control, I will confess: "Lord, Psalm 40 says that when I wait for you that you hear my cry. You bring me out of what feels like a pit and establish me."

_____

_____

_____

Remain in the atmosphere of thanking Him for the work He is doing until the trigger is gone. You may need to revisit worksheets on lies, roots, or shame if the triggers continue. Just do not give up! When you experience peace, it is a very good indicator that God is at work. Let peace rule your heart. (Colossians 3:15; 2 Thessalonians 3:16)

If the triggers continue with your current health plan, you may need to reexamine your plan and determine if it is appropriate. Ask the Lord if the eating or health plan you are on is the correct path. I would suggest spending time in prayer before choosing a new plan. Don't just jump into something without consulting Him and perhaps getting some wise counsel from someone who understands eating disorders and good nutrition. We would not suggest a person in recovery from alcohol to hang out in a bar and we would not expect a person with a past eating disorder to start a health plan that would be harmful.

The Bible gives us some awesome promises; the following is one of my favorites that I like to hang onto when things get tough! He is always faithful!

Psalm 40:1-3 NKJV

I waited patiently for the Lord; And He inclined to me, And heard my cry. 2 He also brought me up out of a horrible pit, Out of the miry clay, And set my feet upon a rock, And established my steps. 3 He has put a new song in my mouth— Praise to our God; Many will see it and fear, And will trust in the Lord.

Chapter 14 -Eating Disorder Scriptures and Prayer Focus

It is easy to google the words eating disorder and find out all the signs and symptoms. We did not want to recreate work that's already been done. We do, however, want to take a look at some spiritual aspects of some of the patterns and behaviors of those with eating disorders and give some ideas on how to process the patterns.

Hiding food or empty food wrappers.

Hiding food can be a shame-based behavior and can reveal a root of a hidden wound. When receiving healing, the person can ask the Lord to reveal the root of the behavior.   See chapter 6 on shame.

If the reason a person hide's food is comfort-based behavior, there still could be shame there, but it is important to ask the Lord what the root is. Worksheet 5 may help with locating any lies that a person believes that the food will actually produce comfort. You may want to take a look at idolatry and ask the Lord what causes you to seek out food instead of Him.

Rules

Part of the torment of an eating disorder are the rules that one must abide by in order to strive for peace. The following can be an example of how the rules get developed:

A person may see a perceived problem like: "I'm too fat." The solution the person sets in order might be to not eat until they lose a certain amount of weight. Another solution the person with an eating disorder tendency might implement is to set up a punishment or penance for doing certain things that they feel will block their ability to lose the fat. For example, the person may decide that if they eat, they will only eat so many bites. As an incentive or a repercussion, if they go over that specific number of bites, they determine they must do a certain task like workout for a specified length of time or perhaps the penance is to make themselves vomit.

The rule is created and then gets adjusted with each failure or the rule can be adjusted spontaneously for no reason.

Rules can dictate anything from what you eat, how you eat or what needs to be done once the rules are violated. The following are ideas on identifying and dealing with rules:

1. SAY THE RULE OUT LOUD

Often, the rules we hear in our mind sound like good ideas. However, when spoken out loud, the fact that the rules are bad ideas are easier to detect. If you start justifying why you should or should not eat, speak the thought out loud. Don't be ashamed to expose it. If you still can't tell if it's a good idea, ask someone who is free and who can hear from God if it's a good idea or not. More often than not, as you are reciting the rule, you'll know if it was a trick to draw you into eating disorder behavior. (Note: The problem is not that there is a rule, but that the rule is fear or bondage based. If the rule produces torment or a lack of peace, please consider going into prayer about the rule.)

2. RESIST the rule

When you hear the rule, speak out loud and resist it. For example, if the rule or thought comes that you can only eat ice for two days and nothing else, submit yourself to the Lord, resist the voice and command it to leave. **Here is a sample prayer:**

"God, I recognize this is not your voice. I submit my will to yours that my body is the temple of Your spirit. I will not deprive my body for the sake of this voice. I resist this voice and in the name of Jesus who came in the flesh, whatever just said to me, "only eat ice," I command you to shut your mouth and go. Do not return. I am not listening to you."

3. Skewed vision

Those suffering from eating disorders do not typically see themselves or others accurately. A too-skinny girl can see herself as fat. A beautiful young woman can look into the mirror and see an old hag. The nature of this view is self-consuming, which is why we will want to be on the lookout for idolatry. Repenting for believing lies and participating in idolatry can be healing as well as help us to commit a life focused on Jesus instead of self. As we focus on the beauty and truth of Jesus, the lies and false perceptions will be revealed. Skewed views can also be a spiritual issue that is likely rooted in lies and shame. See worksheets 5 on lies and 6 on shame. Also consider asking Jesus to clean your vision and eyes. Command anything that is hindering you from seeing to go in Jesus' name.

Scriptures to recite and know might be:

Psalm 19:14

Psalm 139:1-4

Psalm 146:8

Isaiah 61:1-3

4. Obsession with Eating Disorder movies or websites

It can be compelling to those with eating disorders to watch movies related to the subject. When Amber and Kirstie discussed their own stories, it was interesting to find that they both had shows they watched over and over...completely fascinated with the eating disorder content. While working on this section, they both confessed to collecting pictures of attributes, models, or fits of clothing that they found desirable. They carefully created scrapbooks, posters, and pin boards. The terminology used in the eating disorder community is, "thinspiration." (A collection of things to inspire you to keep doing what you are doing.) On hindsight Kirstie says it was a like a form of lust or coveting.

In addition, there are websites that glorify and celebrate eating disorders and the ability to "do it well." Using food and exercise apps can be a part of the obsession to obtain weight loss. Kirstie maintains she used a variety of apps for tracking her progress. They all performed the same function of recording her food and exercise, but she was fearful that she was undercalculating her calories consumed and overcalculating her calories burned.

The first insight into this symptom is the word obsession. Where there is obsession, there is typically idolatry, pride, and error. When leading someone through healing, it is sometimes prudent for the healing person to renounce the specific movie, television show, apps or website that has them "hooked." It would not hurt to cut off soul ties with those with whom they have bonded on the websites. (If pacts were made with other members, those pacts need to be renounced.)

A prayer of healing might look something like this, "Lord, I repent for my indulgent watching or use of _____. I choose to turn away from this and declare you are my inspiration and my healer. I cut off all ties I made with this _____ and with the following people/characters _____. I renounce every pact that I made that does not glorify You. I ask You to close every door I opened through this access and I command anything that does not glorify God that was attached to this behavior to go in Jesus' name."

Laxatives, Pills, and other life controlling substances

Taking laxatives or other substances to control weight can lead to some serious health issues. The draw/pull to purchase laxatives and other medications for weight loss purposes can be as compelling for a person with an eating disorder as it is for a drug addict who is trying to refuse to take another hit. If you feel yourself being drawn to these substances, perhaps you are experiencing a trigger and need to do worksheet #15. Also, see the chapter on evicting trespassers.

Be aware that when you are shopping or see a medication you have used in the past that you could be triggered. Stop what you are doing; pray and let Holy Spirit guide you. He may instruct you to leave the store, call an accountability person, say a scripture, or something else that will turn the temptation into a victory!

Researching Eating Disorders

It is possible to have an eating disorder and not realize it. There are those who have found themselves researching disorders and learning about them and even feeling sorry for those who had issues but were blinded to their own twisted thinking.

If you find yourself seeking for the next big fad diet to try, or researching the latest weight loss medication, you may want to seek the Lord for the truth as to why you are researching.

Sample prayer: Lord, help me to see me like you do. Remove any blindness I have to my own issues and help me to see the truth. I submit myself to You for guidance, healing, and deliverance, if needed.

Web of Connection

When a person with an eating disorder is making a decision to eat something considered taboo, there is more going on in the head than one might imagine. Every decision can be interlocked with a chain of events. A decision of what to eat can be fearful and overwhelming because they aren't just thinking of eating, let's say, a cookie. They look at the cookie and the chain of events weighs heavy. It doesn't necessarily have to be logical. The thought process could look something like this: "She wants me to have a cookie. If I eat that cookie, I will have to hide to purge it when no one is around. That will make me sick. I know I should not have the cookie, so if I eat it, I will have to exercise for three hours to fix it. My leg will start to fidget, I will feel ashamed, and everyone will be thinking how fat I am. I will not want anyone to see me at school and…"

With this string of interlocking web-like scenarios with every decision it is easy to be overloaded and overwhelmed.

When trying to convince a person with an eating disorder to break a rule, we need to remember that there may be a web of connection going on that is not logical. The hurting person can respond with anger or even aggressive behavior. If you are that person who starts to feel aggressive, confused or overwhelmed when someone mentions breaking a rule or makes it impossible for you to follow through with penance or consequences, take note and consider that there is a problem. We know this is torment to you and you need Jesus to heal this area in your life.

Have you ever used a computer and it got bogged down with too much information coming in all at once? Perhaps it gets stuck and you have to reboot it to get it to function. Know that when a person is caught in a mind web, it slows down the processing and is frustrating and overwhelming. A well-meaning person can present the truth, but unless Christ intervenes at that moment, it can be quite difficult to believe the truth or even process it. But, there is hope!

Here are a couple of ideas to deal with the web of connection:

1. Ask Jesus to clear your thought process and remove the tangling/webbing. It is likely you will not be able to do the worksheets until this overwhelming thought process calms down. It is best if you can pray as soon as the tangling begins.
2. Be persistent in letting Jesus do the work to untangle the thought. If a ball of yarn was all tangled, up, you'd have to be persistent in getting it all unknotted. Pray in the fruit of patience and faithfulness!
3. Begin to encourage yourself. Quote the scripture that you can do all things in Christ. (Philippians 4:13) The Bible also says to put on the garment of praise for the spirit of heaviness. (Isaiah 61:3) Begin to pull your mind from the circle of thoughts and fill your mind with gratitude. A great scripture to say to yourself is to confess Philippians 4:8. Here's how to do that:
   — I refuse to think about _____. I will think about what is true, what is noble and whatever is just. I will think on what is just and pure. My mind will be filled with what is lovely and a good report. Lord, help me to meditate on your goodness. I refuse with my will to think about things that do not glorify You!
4. It can be therapeutic to write down all your thoughts and feelings whether it's making a chart, drawing a picture, journaling, painting, or whatever you need to do to get out the emotions. After you do that, offer all of it to Jesus and submit it to Him for truth and healing.
5. Speak the web of thoughts to someone you trust who doesn't struggle with an eating disorder. Let them speak truth into your life, and rest in that truth.

Paranoia

Mood swings, surges of high energy to fatigue laden depression can be a sad part of an eating disorder. Paranoia and distrust rob its victims of peace. It is not unusual for those with eating disorders to spend time weighing and adjusting their food on scales even though the packaging clearly identifies the information. Obsession with the serving size becomes a torment.

An 8th grader started public school for the first time this year. She reported to her mother that she sat for a little while at lunch with girls involved in the school's dance team. It came as a shock to her that the girls did not eat lunch. They discussed among themselves how to adjust food so that they did not gain weight. They were obsessed with how to not eat. The girls did not trust what was given to them and it is unlikely that the parents are even aware of the drive their babies already have to treat food like the enemy.

The root of paranoia could be lies. If you find yourself paranoid or acting out in uncontrollable mania or even depression, the lies worksheet is good. However, we cannot stress the importance of evicting any trespasser. As a believer in Christ, you have the authority to command the enemy to go. No, the enemy does not play fair and we do not need to take one ounce of torment without fighting back and getting our victory! See worksheets 10-12.

Once more, we also want to put a disclaimer that this book is not intended to be a substitute for good medical and mental health care. We believe that Jesus is our healer! We also believe that He can use medical professionals to help when needed.

Notes:

Chapter 15 - Conclusion

We know that getting healthy can be hard work. Don't give up. If you keep going, you will get there. Use this book and its resources to fine tune your journey. If you mess up, get up and keep going. Look at the fruit of the spirit again and do not neglect to pray in the fruit and tend its orchard.

You did not begin this journey of good health in the flesh, if you are following the pattern for freedom in this book. You began looking at your spiritual needs. As Amber and I are finishing up this book, we both have been having some difficulty progressing. Currently, I have lost 113 pounds and have about 42 pounds to go. Amber has lost 60 pounds and only has 10 more pounds to reach her goal weight. During prayer this morning, I thought, "Lord, I do not know how to stay on track. I do not want to go backwards or stall." The following scripture came to mind:

Galatians 3:3 NKJV

Are you so foolish? Having begun in the Spirit, are you now being made perfect by the flesh?

I was reminded that it isn't by sure will power that I'm going to have optimum health and consistent success. I asked the Lord to grow me in the fruit of the spirit and renew my mind. I talked with Amber and she too is going back to some of the precepts we taught in this book. Seek the Lord and all His righteousness first and all things will be added to you! (Matthew 6:3)

If this book has stirred interest in eating disorders, we caution you to take care in looking up eating disorder information online. Even programs that proclaim that they are Christian based can be tainted with non-Biblical beliefs and practices.

We will continue to provide resources on the website: DriveToBeFree.org

Some of the articles and videos you will find on the website are:

- Parenting a child with an eating disorder (See Appendix A for parenting information as well.)
- Signs that your child has an eating disorder
- Testimonies
- Practical tips for staying the course
- Interviews with Lisa, Amber, Kirstie and the River health teams

You would not have made it this far in this work if the Lord had not been leading and guiding you through this process and into victory. It is our prayer, hope and confidence that the Lord Jesus will complete this good work that He has begun in you. (Philippians 1:6)

Our heart's desire is that you prosper in all things and be in health, just as your soul prospers. (3 John 1:2) You can do it. You can be the healthiest version of you. We pray you are not only desperate but driven to be free. Jesus came to this earth for those who are humble enough to know they need a physician. The woman with the issue of blood in Matthew 9:20 was driven with faith and need to press through the crowd. Jesus immediately knew she had touched his clothes. Know this: He responds to those who touch Him with faith and desperation.

The final worksheet is designed to be a praise report. In Luke 17:11-19, we read of 10 lepers who were miraculously healed. Only 1 of those healed men returned to thank their healer. As a result, that one was not only healed but made whole! It is important to give the Lord praise and recognize his goodness. We are so confident that He is doing a great work in you that we want to allow room to praise Him and also provide you with a historical record of the benefits you experience as you make your way to freedom from food and victory in your health!

Worksheet 15 – Praise Report

This worksheet is designed to help you remember all of the great things the Lord does in and for you. When the enemy makes accusations that God hasn't done anything, use this sheet to pray and thank the Lord for everything He has done! Include changes in mindset, any healings in your body, victories over the flesh, body changes, etc.!

What it was like before:	Benefits of what God has done in me:

RESOURCES

We are so glad you have reached this section of your journey into freedom and victory! We have developed companion material to this book to help provide you with support and more information on the topic of freedom including:

- Small Group Curriculum
- Helpful teaching videos and testimonies
- Workshops, Seminars and Retreats
- www.DrivenToBeFree.org

We are in no way affiliated with Mercy Multiplied, but we believe that this residential program does a good work and is a great place for women with life controlling issues like eating disorders, addictions, or areas of brokenness. There are other residential programs we looked into for the resource section of this book, but were hard pressed to find programs which did not include yoga, and certain types of meditation more conducive to new age or religions that are not in harmony with the Holy Bible.

Mercy Multiplied: Mercy is a 6 Month resident program for women ages 13-32 with life controlling issues. https://mercymultiplied.com/

Mercy Multiplied offers helpful books you can purchase or download their free Ebooks. Look for the titles: Starved & Beyond Staved at https://store.mercymultiplied.com/collections/books

We want to stress once more that this book is not intended to replace or give any counsel on medical issues. Having an eating disorder can be a serious and even life-threatening issue. Please take care of yourself and those you love. It is our hope that this book will help you connect with your creator to help you heal and guide you into perfect truth.

APPENDIX A Eating Disorders – Note to Parents

It is difficult to consider that something might be wrong with your child. I was close to my daughter; yet, I did not recognize what I know now were evident signs that she was indeed suffering from the symptoms of an eating disorder.

I am going to provide you with a list of things a parent can look for when considering an eating disorder as a possible issue. However, just because you see these behaviors, it does not necessarily mean that your child has or will develop an eating disorder. Just in case there is an issue, I want to mention something important!

The word Nervosa in Anorexia Nervosa and Bulimia Nervosa means "nervous" in Latin. According to Urban Dictionary, Nervosa has "come to be associated with a behavior, belief or habit that affects the body via the nervous system or the mind." Eating disorders are trauma or stressed induced. My daughter has told me, "There are reasons why a person may have an eating disorder. However, the eating disorder is not the volcano, it is the smoke." It is the fruit, not the root.

The volcano is the root issues and if you take the cap off a volcano, it is going to spew. If you are going to address the smoke, it is wise to expect the lava and pray about how to address this. Those tormented with eating disorders need patience, love, understanding, truth, and kindness.

The world of eating disorders has its own culture. It has its own language, symbols, and thought processes. Know the signs, symptoms and indicators. When I sat down with Kirstie and Amber in the *Driven To Be Free from Food Addictions and Eating Disorders* project, I was amazed and dumbfounded as they discussed the culture of the eating disorder community. Much of what is listed below, I learned from listening to those two compare their own stories. Their research and knowledge of the topic is amazing.

While the content of our book is not a substitute for medical treatment, we do believe that the workbook may help guide a person through processing the "volcano." Eating disorders are serious and need to be treated with wisdom and care. There are a couple of URL links that give more details on medical treatment at the end of this paper.

Lastly, I want to mention that most of those with eating disorders are extremely intelligent even though their thinking is affected greatly or twisted by the proverbial volcano and the smoke. What we are dealing with isn't ignorance as much as it is the results of unhealed trauma, inner wounds, and unchallenged believed lies. – Lisa D. Piper

According to the Society for Adolescent Medicine:

- Eating disorders, such as anorexia, is the third most chronic illness in adolescent females (in terms of time they are sick).
- Eating disorders occur in both boys and girls.

Possible Eating Disorder Indicators:

Shame based behavior:

- Ashamed to eat in front of people
- Ashamed of the amounts of food eaten
- Avoiding mirrors, activities where people will see their body
- Hiding food, wrappers, or evidence of having eaten
- Disgust or self-hate towards body or weight
- Hiding behind bulky clothes

Obsessive behaviors:

- Obsessing over:
    - Calories, fats, carbs
    - Dieting and fad diets
    - Vomiting, Laxatives, diuretics, diet pills
    - Photos of thin "perfect" looking bodies or body parts
        - Photos can include anything from an entire person, or specific areas that depict thinness such as clavicles, rib cages, or thigh gaps.
    - Thinspiration/Thin-Inspiration boards or journals to hold photos or clippings that focus on desired physical goals
    - Exercising
    - Movies or books with eating disorder content
    - Measuring or Weighing Self
    - Measuring or weighing foods
        - Often the person will overestimate weight or calories to make sure they do not go over. For example, if a handful of almonds weigh 2 ounces, they may record 2.5 ounces.

- o Trying on clothing over and over again
- o Specific Ways to eat food or how much to eat: Food Rituals
  - ▪ In one video, Amber talks about only eating a popsicle to the wooden stick. Kirstie talks about eating only the top part of the upper part of a bagel. Perhaps a food ritual is eating only 8 pecans or cutting bread into certain kinds of pieces before consuming.
- o Overachieving or Perfectionism

Frustration or feeling overwhelmed:

- A person with an eating disorder may feel frustrated, agitated, upset, or overwhelmed when:
  - o Making food-related choices, especially if they are unprepared
  - o Unable to figure out how to go purge
    - ▪ If they are made to eat, their mind may go into overdrive on how they are going to hide and purge. The fear can be so great that they may avoid eating just because they do not know how they can get rid of what they've ingested.
  - o Asked to go out to eat or told to eat something that they deem unacceptable
  - o Given a menu and asked to pick out a food
    - ▪ There can be a lot of chatter going on in the mind. When the shame, guilt, chatter, and outside stimuli all collide, it can be overwhelming.
  - o There is no control of what is being consumed
  - o Told a food has a certain calorie count, but then feel as if they've been given false information

Perception & Behaviors:

- Fear of being overweight
- Does not see oneself as thin, even if underweight
- Approach eating disorder topics with care. If there is an eating disorder present, the person will likely deny this or can become hostile when approached
- Difficulty concentrating or sleeping

- Adolescents who become vegetarians may do so in order to avoid eating certain foods and thereby avoid questions from adults as to why they are not eating.
- There may be food texture issues involved with an eating disorder.
  - One girl completely avoided custard-type textures. Once she tasted the texture, a binge immediately followed.
- Self-hate. Speaks words of hating certain body parts or loathing appearance. May be unable to look in the mirror without grimacing.
- Depressed/Moody
- Fear of not being able to stop eating while bingeing
- Anxiety

OTHER INDICATORS:

- Irregular periods or no period at all (when there is no other explanation)
- The body may try to heat itself up by growing fine body hair called lanugo
- Scarring on the back of the fingers from self-induced throwing up
- It can be very painful to take the number of laxatives that a person with an eating disorder may take. This is not a fun issue. However, some describe that when the medicine has done its work, they feel clean. Perhaps those who vomit after eating have this euphoria as well. One woman described it as follows:
  - "it does not make sense. I know it doesn't make sense to take laxatives. Even scientific studies show it doesn't cause weight loss, it just makes a person dehydrated, but I was drawn and compelled to do it even though I hated it. The elated clean feeling at the end was my reward. I did not know that what I was experiencing was bondage. The drive to do what I did was overwhelming. I am free of that now, but I remember what it was like. The clean feeling was a lie. It never stayed. Having an eating disorder was like having a false protector. As long as I focused on the eating disorder and its issues, I did not have to look deeper at what was causing it. In a very weird sense, the focus on the food just kept me too busy to deal with the real problems."

Media & Social Indicators:

Check social media and websites for:

- Eating disorder sites or activity in pro eating disorder groups or websites.
  - (There are communities who encourage one another in being the best at anorexia, bulimia or purging.)
  - Sites that promote:
    - ED (eating disorder), Ana (short for anorexia)
    - Mia (short for bulimia)
    - EDNOS (eating disorders not otherwise specified)
  - Verbiage/language used in eating disorder communities:
    - Ana, Mia, or Ed are not names of online friends. They represent different variations of the disorder. Even the name Deb can refer to depression.
    - These communities can be proud of their disorder, they do not believe anything is wrong and may boast about their exploits like eating 100 calories a day or exercising for an unhealthy period of time.

Spiritual note: Soul ties can be created with these communities and need to be renounced and severed. In addition, these tight communities are tied together with a bond and can produce rebellion, pride, and twisted thinking. We cover this in chapter 13 of *Driven to Be Free from Food Addictions and Eating Disorders*

Symbols and Community Signs:

NOTE: Just because your child is wearing one of these symbols does not mean that it represents an eating disorder. They could just like the color or symbol and not know what it may represent.

- **Pro Ana means to be in favor of anorexia.** There are communities online who unite and embrace their eating disorder. They may be focused on becoming skinnier or "staying healthy".
- **Pro Mia means to be in favor of bulimia.** There are also communities who come together to embrace this disorder. Be careful in what websites are permissible. Some Websites may advertise that they are created to support those with eating disorders,

but upon looking deeper, they offer sources for reinforcing disordered behaviors. Often, the information on these sites glorify unhealthy bodies, and equip members (via forums) to give each other ideas on how to be better at their eating disorder.

Kids find acceptance and inclusion in what can prove to be deadly practices. Many members of Pro-ED communities believe that eating disorders are a lifestyle "choice" and not a disorder. As outlined in the book, *Driven to be Free from Food Addictions and Eating Disorders*, these thought processes are twisted and even when addressed, the person may not receive the fact that they are not thinking correctly.

- **Pro Ana symbols:** The bracelets are thin and red and often have a dragonfly charm or clasp. Wearing the bracelet is a sign of acceptance of the disorder. The bracelet is often worn on the left wrist.
- **Pro Mia symbols:** The bracelets are blue or purple and often worn on the right wrist. They may also have a butterfly clasp or charm. The bracelets may have beads, may be purchased or handmade.
- **Custom symbols:** Some advocates may combine the symbols or colors to make their own custom jewelry.
- **Self-harm bracelet:** Those involved in self-harm communities may wear a black beaded bracelet.
- **The bracelets serve the following purposes:**
  1. Identification to other community members
  2. Reminders to not eat
  3. Encouragement for others in the community
  4. Acceptance of the eating disorder and their community

Other Symbols of Note:

The symbol to the left is used as the symbol that denotes: Eating Disorder Recovery

The semi-colon has become a symbol for suicide. This is meant to raise awareness, but under twisted thinking, a person may use this symbol as a "badge of honor."

The following information is from Lucile Packard Children's Hospital Stanford:

"Many physical symptoms linked to anorexia are often due to starvation and malnourishment. They may include:

- ✓ Belly pain
- ✓ Constipation
- ✓ Lethargy
- ✓ Fluid loss (dehydration)

- ✓ Extreme tiredness (fatigue)
- ✓ Sensitivity to cold temperatures
- ✓ Being abnormally thin (emaciated)

- ✓ Dizziness
- ✓ Growth of fine, downy body hair (lanugo)
- ✓ Yellowing of the skin
- ✓ Very dry skin (when pinched and let go, it stays pinched)

These symptoms may seem like other health problems. Have your child see his or her healthcare provider for a diagnosis. Early diagnosis and treatment are vital and can help prevent future problems.